THE BETTER BIRTH BOOK

THE BETTER BIRTH BOOK

*Taking the Mystery (and Fear)
Out of Childbirth*

Tracy Donegan

The Liffey Press

Published by
The Liffey Press
Ashbrook House, 10 Main Street,
Raheny, Dublin 5, Ireland
www.theliffeypress.com

A catalogue record of this book is
available from the British Library.

ISBN 1-904148-87-5

Printed in the Republic of Ireland by ColourBooks Ltd.

CONTENTS

ABOUT THE AUTHOR

Tracy Donegan is a Certified Doula, HypnoBirthing® educator and mother. Born in Dublin, Tracy has lived abroad for the past 12 years, most recently in Singapore. She has recently returned to Dublin to establish the first doula service in Ireland. Passionate about birth and its effects on both the mother and newborn, Tracy also runs the Irish chapter of the International Caesarean Awareness Network, a support group for anyone negatively affected by an unplanned caesarean.

Acknowledgements

A sincere thank you to everyone who has encouraged me to write (and re-write) this book. I'm very grateful to the many mothers of Ireland who have shared their birth stories, insights and experiences with me, and allowed me to share them with you. Although many experts provided assistance on this book, the real experts are the mothers who are once again listening to the wisdom of their own birthing instincts and bringing their babies into this world gently and confidently. To my family, who have shared this journey with me, especially my son Jack who, unbeknownst to him, planted the seeds of this book when he was born in March 2003. A special thank you to my husband Philip, the best father a son could have. I am indebted to the following for advice, inspiration and permission to publish some of their insights: Dr Michel Odent; Sheila Kitzinger; Andrea Robertson; Janelle Durham; Marsden Wagner; Sheila Stubbs; Hazel Larkin; Dr Sarah J. Buckley; Laura Shanley; Patricia Newton; Maternity Center Association; Center for Improvements in Maternity Services; Ginny Phang; Jock Doubleday; Skylar Browning; Cuidiu (Irish Childbirth Trust); Dr Paul Tseng; Dr F. M. Lai; and Janet Tamaro. Thanks also to the people behind the following websites for permission to reproduce and adapt some of their work: www.birthlove.com; www.sarahjbuckley.com; www.aims.org.uk; www.mothering.com; www.birthpsychology.com; www.birthinternational.com, and all other websites and sources credited in the text.

To the Midwives of Ireland

"Courage doesn't always roar. Sometimes courage is the quiet voice at the end of the day saying, 'I will try again tomorrow.'"
— Mary Anne Radmacher

INTRODUCTION

WHY THIS BOOK?

Why should you read this book? Simple really: if you are having a baby in Ireland, you want to know about Irish maternity care. Shelves in bookshops are straining under the weight of books on pregnancy and birth, but almost all written from a US or UK perspective. Irish women have told me again and again that they want a book written by an Irish woman for Irish women. So here it is!

Being pregnant is a wonderful experience for most of us. (Of course, we're all guilty of indulging in a little griping now and then!) But how can you really take the time to enjoy pregnancy when you have so many decisions to make? Plus, it seems like the closer the big day looms, the more decisions you have — *and* you're on a deadline that keeps moving! *The Better Birth Book* answers the questions you have and more importantly those you never even thought to ask, so you can make the best choices for you *and* your baby.

We are bombarded with opinions and studies about pregnancy and birth. We hear reports on the news, we read about it online, we get tons of unsolicited advice from our friends and relatives. What or whom should we believe? How can we make sense of it all, especially when faced with important decisions that can have lasting effects on ourselves and our children? Years ago, the biggest decision you had to make was what colour to paint the baby's room! Now, it's "public or private?"; "home or hospital?"; "midwife or consultant?"; "epidural or natural?"; "kneeling or squatting?" . . . you get the picture.

So where do you even begin? Well, let's start with the star of the show: your new baby. There has always been a lot of focus on the mother's experience and how different choices can affect her. It's only very recently that science has started to look at the baby's experience of pregnancy and birth. Once you bring your baby into the decision-making, then that mountain of choices you have to make becomes much more manageable. Now, unless you have an exceptionally gifted baby that can do Morse code on your organs (kicking your bladder for "yes" and your ribs for "no") it's quite difficult to get your baby's views on anything! So how do you know what is best for your baby? You will want to be sure that every choice you make is based on sound research (i.e. backed by science) so that any medical choice — whether it's antenatal testing, birth positions, drugs, etc. — is made on the basis of real medical indications. It should not just be something that is done routinely for everybody. Throughout the book, I have attempted to indicate in plain English what the latest and best research says about a particular option you have.

FEAR-FREE BIRTH

There are two kinds of realities: factual reality (supported by science) and perceived reality (your beliefs, and/or your caregiver's beliefs) It is a *fact* that in the western world around 80 to 90 per cent of mothers will have normal pregnancies and give birth between 37 and 42 weeks without any problems. But the *perceived* reality for many women is that birth is a disaster waiting to happen. It doesn't matter what science tells us if we believe otherwise. Our beliefs have been formed throughout our childhood and teenage years and won't just change overnight. Most mothers believe that our bodies are destined to fail and have forgotten the *fact* that we've been having babies for millions of years. It is a *myth* that birth became safer once it was moved to the hospital. Science tells us that, for low-risk pregnancies (most of you reading this book), home birth is in fact the better option — and yet our hospitals are still full every day of mothers with low-risk pregnancies. Facing our fears means we have to ask ourselves: Is this fear a factual reality (supported by science and best evidence) or is it my perception?

Another reason for writing this book is to dispel much of the fear and many of the myths that seem to surround pregnancy these days. When did pregnancy get to be such a worrying and fearful time? Whatever happened to blissfully happy mums-to-be? Our instant information age probably has a lot to do with it. You just have to log on to any pregnancy chat room or forum and instead of chatting with expectant mothers, you're bombarded with topics such as "stabbing pains", "c-section scar infection", "swollen fingers", "my baby is too small", "my baby is too big", "I'm anaemic", "I'm not anaemic" . . . No doubt you've heard that if you have morning sickness, then that "proves" that baby is doing fine — it's the "hormones" . . . but if you're one of those women who are lucky enough *not* to have morning sickness (or, as some call it, morning, noon and night sickness), then you worry yourself to death for a few weeks wishing you would throw up! How ridiculous is that?!

While I could blame the internet for all of this scary information, daytime TV doesn't exactly help. In these shows, we'll innocently follow a cheerful woman talking about her forthcoming "event" — and then cut to the birth where they say something like, "Will Claire and her baby survive? We'll find out right after this break!" Such suspense works fine for *The X-Factor,* but for a show about birth?! So, of course, we're all glued to our seats, thinking, "If it can happen to Claire, it could happen to me" when, in fact, most pregnancies are low risk. You've heard the horror stories from family and friends over the years. When was the last time you heard a positive birth story? Doctors themselves are also guilty of projecting their own beliefs or perceptions rather than the statistical realities.

So despite the "risky" tests, the possible perils of filling your car with petrol or eating mayonnaise with your ham sandwich, the recklessness of drinking a caffeinated beverage or having a sip of wine at a wedding, the odds are overwhelmingly in a pregnant woman's favour that, around 40 weeks or so from conception, one way or another and mostly regardless of what she has or hasn't done, the average pregnant woman will give birth and her baby will be just fine. Talk to women who have recently "passed over" to motherhood and they'll tell you that they wish they had spent a lot more time sleeping than worrying about whether or not they should have eaten that tuna sandwich for lunch. They'll also tell you to relax and enjoy your pregnancy (swollen ankles and all) because you only get one chance to carry your little bundle of joy this close to you, all to yourself, for the rest of her life and yours.

HOW TO USE THIS BOOK

This book is intended as a guide to the experience of labour and childbirth. Much of what you read in these pages will differ from what you usually hear in hospital antenatal classes or read about in the mainstream pregnancy magazines. My hope is that after reading it, you may question some of your own beliefs about birth and maybe get a glimpse of how wonderful birth and becoming a new mum can be.

There is a *huge* amount of information available on pregnancy and birth. Sometimes, this can be truly bewildering. I have made use of some of the best available resources to bring to you the latest and best evidence on everything from how make informed choices about the type of care you receive, to complementary therapies, to pain relief in labour. Look out for shaded boxes to guide you through these issues. And there are simple, practical tips that you can use to deal with everything from home birth to getting your baby into the best position for birth to breastfeeding. For these practical tips, just look out for the following little picture:

There is a glossary on pages 236–241 to explain some of the more unfamiliar terms (and some that you may be familiar with). In the text, I have highlighted terms that are explained in the glossary, usually on their first use, by writing them in **bold print**, and by this little picture in the margin:

Simple! If only figuring out your maternity benefit were as easy But don't worry, we cover that in Appendix B, along with other government guidelines on rights and entitlements. And Appendix A provides information on hospital policies and statistics on some of the issues and choices discussed in the book, to help guide you towards the form of care that you feel suits you best.

As this is a book about birth I have only touched on pregnancy. Some great books on pregnancy are:

- *Pregnancy and Childbirth* by Sheila Kitzinger

- *The Pregnancy Book* by Sears and Sears

- *Pregnancy, Childbirth and the Newborn* by Penny Simkin

- *Having a Baby Naturally* by Peggy O'Mara

These and other books of interest are listed at the back of the book.

Throughout the book I have included actual birth stories to illustrate what a momentous event birth is in our lives, and how every birth is different. (I have changed names and some details to preserve privacy.) What will your birth story be? My hope is that your birth story will be one of excitement and empowerment — the excitement of those first labour twinges and the empowerment of being informed and confidently making the right choices for you and your baby.

In fact, I want to end this introduction with a highly unusual, but incredibly empowering birth story from the US — unusual in the sense that it shows that it is possible to have a fear-free, pain-free birth experience. Laura Shanley is the mother of four children, all born at home without the help of doctors or midwives. Laura's husband, David, caught their first baby and Laura herself caught the other three. Neither of them had been trained in midwifery or medicine. Today, the Shanleys teach other women their methods. Perhaps one day a birth story such as theirs will not be so unusual . . .

DO-IT-YOURSELF CHILDBIRTH

By Laura Shanley

Prepare to be amazed: I had an unassisted conception. My husband and I closed the bedroom door, took off our clothes, and conceived a child without any help from anyone! David got an erection without drugs of any sort, and actually proceeded to impregnate me without consulting a manual or consultant.

Even more amazing is that I didn't have a conception coach! No one stood next to the bed shouting "Push! Push! Pant! Pant!" Somehow, I just knew what to do!

Are you shocked? Are you impressed? Probably not. This is because the majority of babies in the world have been safely conceived this way throughout all of eternity. So why are you amazed when I say that I also had an unassisted pregnancy and birth?

"Well," you say, "because conception is easy, but pregnancy and birth are not." I beg to differ. Pregnancy is a natural, healthy condition. It is not a disease. If a woman is physically and psychologically healthy, there is absolutely no need to measure her tummy, test her urine, or check her blood. Needles hurt because skin is not designed to be punctured.

Even if a woman isn't healthy, does she really need a "professional" to inform her of the fact? Are women totally incapable of determining the state of their own health? And suppose they aren't healthy. Can a "professional" actually *make* them well? Perhaps if they believe in the professional more than they believe in themselves. I believe I am my own best caregiver. I have much more faith in my own abilities than I've ever had in any doctor or midwife.

Childbirth — the word alone makes most people cringe. Instantly, one imagines a frightened, tearful woman lying in a hospital bed surrounded by masked men and women and perhaps a family member. Monitors are beeping and people are yelling "PUSH! PUSH!" as the poor woman struggles with all her might to expel her baby. Her forehead is sweating and periodically she cries, "I can't do this anymore!" Medical personnel assure her that she can — but if she can't, they will be more than happy to assist her with drugs, forceps, scissors and a knife, if necessary. Thank God for modern medicine. How did we ever survive without it?

The truth is, we did survive and can continue to survive, quite well in most cases, especially when it comes to giving birth. First, however, we must rid ourselves of the belief that childbirth is a painful, dangerous ordeal that must always be supervised and assisted by "skilled professionals". I chose to believe otherwise, and this is my story.

I first became interested in childbirth when I was about six years old. After listening to my mother's explanation of what actually happens in birth, however, my interest was short lived. "After they shave you, the doctor makes a little cut to make more room for the baby," she said. That's all I needed to hear. If there were to be any children in my future, someone else was going to have to give birth to them.

Changing Perceptions

As I grew older, movies and television helped fill in all the gory details. Obviously, I reasoned, pregnancy was a disease complete with vomiting, backaches, swollen ankles and strange cravings. If you survived it, you could look forward to hours or maybe days of excruciating labour pains, followed by weeks in the hospital. Motherhood was becoming increasingly unappealing.

My perception of childbirth changed, however, when at the age of 18 my husband-to-be, David, presented me with a copy of Grantly Dick-Read's *Childbirth Without Fear*. Dick-Read was an English physician who used chloroform to ease labour pains, as was the custom in the first half of the twentieth century. But one night, something happened that forever changed his perception of birth.

He went to the house of a poor countrywoman who was about to have a child. When he felt the birth was near, he offered her the chloroform, but the woman refused to take it. This was the first time he had ever seen a woman refuse it, and yet the woman remained perfectly calm and the baby was born easily. As he was leaving, he asked her why she had chosen to give birth without an anaesthetic and she replied, "It didn't hurt. It wasn't meant to, was it, doctor?"

Over the next few years, Dick-Read encountered other women who appeared to have little or no pain in childbirth. What, he wondered, could explain why some women suffered and others did not. He went on to study it extensively. He discovered that the women who suffered the most in childbirth were the ones who were most afraid.

Fear, he learned, has a profound effect on the body. When a person is in a state of fear, messages are sent to the body telling it to either fight the perceived danger or run away from it. Blood and oxygen instantly rush into the muscle structure, which in turn gives the body the power it needs to survive. Any organs that are not needed for either "fight or flight" are consequently drained of blood (and oxygen) so that it may be diverted elsewhere. This explains why people turn "white as a sheet" when they're afraid. The body assumes that the face is not in need of blood and oxygen as much as the legs, for instance, which when given the extra "fuel", enable the endangered person to run.

In addition to the face, blood is also drained from the brain, the digestive organs and the uterus. Dick-Read found that the uterus of a frightened woman in labour is literally white. Without the fuel it needs, the uterus cannot function correctly, nor can waste products be carried away. Therefore, labour hurts. The solution — eliminate the fear and you eliminate the pain.

Dick-Read's theories made sense to me. Maybe childbirth wouldn't be so bad after all, I thought. Less than two years later, David and I moved in together and I got the chance to see for myself.

In addition to *Childbirth Without Fear*, we had also been reading other books that dealt with how our beliefs create our reality. Little by little, we were beginning to create the life we desired. Why, we wondered, shouldn't we be able to create the birth we desired, as well? In November 1977, I conceived.

Everyday I repeated my belief suggestions, "I believe in my ability to give birth safely and easily at home," I told myself. "I believe I'm not afraid, I believe I'm safe, I believe I'm innocent. I believe I'm deserving of a good birth." I examined every aspect of my consciousness, looking for any beliefs that might prevent me from having the kind of birth I desired. I also practised giving birth frequently in my dreams.

Consequently, I had almost none of the so-called symptoms of pregnancy. I vomited only one day, and that stopped when I realised I still had some fears about becoming a mother. "I'm not afraid of being a mother," I told myself, and I never vomited again.

I went into labour on the afternoon of 20 August 1978. The contractions weren't completely painless, but they weren't anything that I couldn't easily handle. Around midnight, David and I called up three of our friends who had asked to attend, along with a filmmaker who wanted to film the birth. Within a half an hour, everyone was there, and we proceeded to talk and laugh and generally enjoy ourselves. We didn't time contractions or check to see how dilated I was. We simply relaxed, had fun, and trusted that when the time was right, the baby would be born.

At about 1.30 am, my water bag broke and I reached down and felt the baby's face. I walked over to the bed, got on my hands and knees, and was about to turn over when I heard an inner voice say, "Don't turn over." I didn't, and a second later my beautiful baby boy, John, literally flew into David's hands. The birth had been a tremendous success. Fifteen months later, I conceived my second son, Willie, and also delivered him, feet first, at home into my own hands. Eighteen months after having Willie, I conceived my daughter, Joy.

This time I thought I might like to be alone for the birth. I had come to trust my body completely. On the morning of 17 November 1982, I went into labour. My sons were sleeping and David was at the campus library. I took a shower, got out my little bathtub, and got down on one foot and one knee, the position that felt right to me this time. When I felt her head crowning, I gave one push and she slipped gently into my hands. She looked right up at me and gave a little cry. The thought went through my mind that she was the most beautiful gift I had ever received.

After cutting the cord, wrapping her in a blanket and delivering the placenta into the bathtub, I went over to the couch to lie down. Soft bells and the sound of ocean waves filled my head. I felt positively blissful. An hour or two later, I got up and took a shower. Then Joy, John, Willie, a friend of mine and I all walked over to the campus to see David. The temperature was in the 70s and I felt as if I were floating on air. This, I thought, is how birth is supposed to be.

A Relaxed Birth

My last child, Michelle, was born on 5 April 1987. That morning I awoke feeling mild contractions. David was up reading the paper, but I decided not to tell him that I was in labour. As I lay in my bed, I breathed deeply and said belief suggestions. I told myself, "I'm moving out of the way and allowing my body to give birth." Suddenly I felt myself slip into a state of complete relaxation. I had absolute faith that the consciousness within me that knew how to grow my baby perfectly, also knew how to get my baby out. My job was simply to relax and allow it to happen.

An hour later, I decided to get up and take a bath. I walked across the hall, turned on the bath water and sat down on the toilet. As I looked between my legs, I saw my water bag beginning to protrude. It popped, I gave a little push, and my little girl slipped into my hands. "David," I called out, "will you come here a minute?"

David came down the hall and was amazed to see Michelle sitting on my lap, peacefully nursing. "You'd better find a scissors," I said, "and turn off the bath water, please."

My story is not unique. Throughout history, women have given birth successfully without medical assistance. In fact, the infant mortality rate in this country rose sharply after women began giving birth in hospitals. Even today, numerous studies show that for the majority of women, home birth is actually safer than hospital birth.

Childbirth is a natural process, which works best when it is interfered with least. Or, as Grantly Dick-Read writes, "If left alone in labour, the body of a woman produces most easily the baby that is not interfered with by its mother's mind or the assistant's hand."

Most childbirth "professionals", however, those whose income and self-esteem are dependent upon women turning themselves over to the "authorities" in labour, would have us believe otherwise. The truth is, with the proper beliefs, any woman can give birth easily, either by herself or in the company of a partner, friends or family. What better place to start believing in our own abilities than with the birth of a child?

© Laura Shanley. Adapted and reproduced with kind permission
of the author. www.ucbirth.com

You're Pregnant!
What Now?

There's a line — mother of God, there's a line!!!

This is usually a time of great excitement and terror . . . and excitement . . . and more terror! *I'm going to be somebody's mother —* that thought scared me more than labour did. Every pregnancy is different, whether it's your first or fifth. It's normal to feel overwhelmed by the news that you're pregnant. You're about to start the job of a lifetime (and you may not have even applied for it). Even if this pregnancy is something you were planning, the realisation of actually being pregnant is like getting on a rollercoaster for the first time; once the ride starts, you're on it until the end. How much you enjoy the ride depends a lot on how you perceive the experience and who is there with you through the twists and turns, ups and downs. If you see pregnancy as being something to look forward to rather than a disruption to your life you'll enjoy the ride a lot more. Above all, keep in mind that pregnancy is temporary. You won't be pregnant forever (although it can feel like that towards the end).

If you think you are pregnant and those ten home pregnancy tests (just to be really really sure) are positive, the first step is usually a visit to your GP, who will do some tests, such as taking your blood and weighing you, and will use the date of your last period to estimate when the baby is due (this is a rough estimate, not an appointment; more on this later). You can discuss with your GP whether you plan to give birth in a hospital or at home, and they may give you some advice on what your best options are. If you go the hospital route, your GP will then provide you with a "letter of referral" to the maternity hospital, if one is needed. If you're planning to have your baby at home, see the chapter on home birth. If you decide on having combined care you can save yourself a lot of time hanging out in the hospital as most of your visits will be with your GP. (See Appendix B, pages 223–226 for more on combined care, public and private care, etc.)

THE FIRST ANTENATAL VISIT

If you are going the hospital route, the first antenatal visit is always such an exciting one — and unfortunately it's usually a long one too. The visit can last about two hours (that may not even include waiting time). By contrast, you could blink and you'd miss your next visit, it'll be so quick, if your pregnancy is normal. Your first hospital visit, to assess your health and your baby's progress, will probably be happen some time between the twelfth and twentieth week. You will probably meet a **midwife**, who will talk to you about your health and answer any concerns you might have. This will also be an opportunity for you to ask about your care and the range of services that are available to you. You will be asked for a urine sample (get used to peeing in a cup — you'll have it down to a fine art by the time your baby is born), will have your blood pressure taken and will have some blood tests. This visit may also involve an **ultrasound** scan, though the first scan is often around 20 weeks.

Once you have met the midwife, she will probably give you a general physical examination, which will assess:

- Your weight;

- The general health of your heart and lungs;

- The size of your baby (an abdominal exam);

- Whether you have any swelling or varicose veins on your hands and legs (excessive swelling can be a symptom of **pre-eclampsia**);

You may also be given the following examinations:

- A smear test and internal exam (not fun but necessary).

- A pelvic examination (to see if your **uterus** is the right size according to your dates).

- Some blood will also be taken to check for your blood type, sexually transmitted diseases, Hep B, your immunity to **rubella** and your rhesus status.

As your pregnancy progresses, you will return at regular intervals for further antenatal visits; you will be asked to bring a urine sample, and your blood pressure will be assessed. Don't be shy about asking any questions that occur to you between visits or during a visit. The only stupid question is the one you don't ask. If you're like me, you might want to write down a few questions as you think of them before each visit — just so you don't look like a rabbit caught in the headlights when your doctor asks, "Any questions?"

ANTENATAL CLASSES

> When our second child was on the way, my wife and I attended an antenatal class aimed at couples that had already had at least one child. The instructor raised the issue of breaking the news to the older child. It went like this: "Some parents," she said, "tell the older child, 'We love you so much we decided to bring another child into this family.' But think about that. Ladies, what if your husband came home one day and said, 'Honey, I love you so much I decided to bring home another wife.'" One of the women spoke up immediately. "Does she cook?"

Antenatal classes in Ireland are designed to introduce mothers-to-be to the world of pregnancy, birth and parenting. Understanding the basic physiology of birth is important for all mothers to understand (although most of us already know that the stork doesn't actually bring the baby). However, surprisingly, the importance of the hormone balance for an easy birth is rarely discussed (see pages 83–85).

Ironically, most antenatal classes focus on coping strategies for the side effects (severe pain and longer labours) that come from disturbing this delicate balance of hormones.

Antenatal classes are also a chance to meet other expectant parents. When everyone at work rolls their eyes when you mention swollen ankles again or, God forbid, the dreaded piles, it's such a treat to have so many sympathisers at the antenatal classes — safety in numbers. While the bulk of the material taught at antenatal classes relates specifically to labour and birth, they can be a great source of practical advice on parenting. Topics covered may include:

- Taking care of your body during pregnancy

- How the foetus develops in utero

- Recognising signs that labour may be starting

- Your options for labour and delivery

- Pain relief

- Possible interventions.

Classes may also cover practical aspects of breastfeeding, parentcraft (everything from changing nappies to holding your baby), childcare, etc.

Antenatal classes are organised by hospitals and independent educators such as Cuidiu (The Irish Childbirth Trust), who are not associated with any particular hospital. They fill up quickly so book your place early. Classes are mostly attended by first-time mothers alone or accompanied by their partners. You will probably attend antenatal classes from about 20 to 30 weeks. Some hospitals are happy to have fathers come along to just one or two of the classes (much to the delight of most Dads). Some hospitals also provide classes for couples with special needs and refresher classes for couples having their second baby. Classes are generally held over six to eight sessions (there are also intensive one day or weekend courses).

Hospital-organised antenatal classes are generally free of charge. There may be benefits to taking antenatal classes run by independent practitioners as you'll get a good overview of the routine procedures and policies in many hospitals and not just the one you are attending. However, these are not free.

DUMB EXCUSES NOT TO TAKE ANTENATAL CLASSES

By Patricia Newton

I think I already know enough between watching television birthing shows and reading

In the eyes of some women, watching television birthing shows regularly is equal to true education. What you may not realise, however, is that what is shown as routine procedures on any particular episode is not necessarily what might occur routinely in the hospital where you will be giving birth. Common interventions vary widely from region to region, and from one caregiver to another.

In addition, because most of these shows are condensed to fit into 30 minutes (including commercials!), you do not see everything that led up to a particular point in any labour. For example, if a woman's labour stalls or stops, there are many reasons why this could happen. There are also several things the woman could try to help speed her labour or get it started again before medical interventions are needed. However, these informative issues are seldom shown or discussed in these shows.

What would be more helpful to you would be to enrol in a good childbirth education class, taught by a professional who is familiar with the common birthing practices in your area. In such a class you would learn the pros and cons of these procedures and be encouraged to discuss any concerns you may have with your own care provider.

As for reading, there are many excellent books available for the pregnant woman. Some of them are *Ina May's Guide to Childbirth* by Ina May Gaskin; *Gentle Birth Choices* by Barbara Harper; *Pregnancy, Childbirth and the Newborn* by Penny Simkin, Janet Whalley and Ann Keppler; and *Mind Over Labour* by Carl Jones.

Mums who have previously given birth say you forget everything you heard in class once that first contraction hits

Any childbirth education class worth your time will teach you many tools you can use during the stages of labour. Some of these tools are deep relaxation, massage, faith, vocalisation, aromatherapy, changing positions, and affirmations. There are many others to learn about as well.

However, being given tools and actually practicing them are two very different things. You might learn of breathing techniques or labouring positions in class, but if you decide not to practise any of the important tools at home, chances are you won't be ready to use them to your advantage once labour begins.

If you are serious about preparing for labour, you will become very familiar with the many things you can do to cope with contractions, shorten your labour and reduce your pain. And if you become familiar with them during pregnancy, you will know how to use them properly during your labour.

On the other hand, if you are not dedicated to practising and preparing, you just might not have a clue how to deal with contractions. But is that the fault of the antenatal teacher?

The nurses are there to help you get through labour

Midwives would love to be able to give you one-to-one continuous support during your labour, but the many demands of their job may not allow them to do this. They are also required to monitor, chart, keep doctors informed of the status of their patients and administer medications. And if they have more than one patient in labour, they have to take care of that patient as well. In addition, midwives have breaks from their shift and there comes a time when their shift ends. Which means they leave and a different midwife is assigned to you.

Although midwives are likely to help you work through contractions for short periods of time, they may not be able to stay beside you and witness every contraction you face. In most cases, they are not someone with whom you already have a bond. Your midwife is usually someone you don't know well, or someone you've never even seen before.

So, skipping the childbirth education class and planning on having a midwife provide continuous labour support for you may not be a realistic plan.

I'd rather spend the money on something for the baby

Yes, independent childbirth education classes do cost money. But spending your money on something for your baby instead of a class that can truly help you have a shorter, easier and safer labour with an end result of a healthier baby comes down to one thing: a matter of priority.

Only you can decide what you think is more important.

Along with pregnancy comes responsibility. Responsible parents make decisions during pregnancy in the best interest of their child. This begins with choosing a medical care provider who is right for them and attending an informative, empowering childbirth education class.

© *Patricia Newton, a leading childbirth educator, lactation educator and doula in Southern New Jersey. www.proudpregnancies.com*

ULTRASOUND SCANS

Your first ultrasound may well be the moment when everything becomes real. You knew you were pregnant, but now you get to see the little person who is turning your world upside down, and you haven't had the pleasure of meeting them yet. It's an emotional moment for many parents. The first scan is usually offered to pregnant women at around 12–14 weeks (sometimes referred to as your early "dating" or "booking" scan). This is when your caregiver will give you your **EDD** (your guess date); early scans are usually more accurate. In certain circumstances, for example, if there are any particular risks or problems, you may be able to have earlier or later scans if necessary.

What Happens During an Ultrasound?

Ultrasound scans use a transducer which sends sound waves through your abdomen to your uterus. The "echoes" it produces are translated by computer into the shapes you can see on the screen — your very first glimpse of your baby!

You will usually be asked to keep your bladder full; this allows for a better reading. A gel is smeared across your abdomen (it's usually freezing; would it kill them to heat it up?) and the midwife or technician moves the transducer around until she can see the baby clearly. She will probably explain to you exactly what you are seeing — heartbeat, hands, legs, head, etc. Ask any questions you want at this stage.

Ultrasound scans can also be carried out using a vaginal probe. This is not very common in Ireland and is more likely to be used if you've had bleeding early on and suspect a miscarriage.

Reasons for Using Ultrasound

Ultrasound scans are mainly used to check:

- What stage your pregnancy is at

- Whether you are carrying one baby or more

- Whether your baby is developing normally

- How well your baby is growing

- The position of the baby and the **placenta** and the level of **amniotic fluid**.

Ultrasound scans are also useful in identifying certain problems, such as bleeding in early pregnancy, growth problems, etc. They can also be used to guide diagnostic tests or operations that may have to be undertaken.

Are Ultrasounds Safe?

There is still some debate around the safety of ultrasounds and the effects on the unborn baby, although most doctors consider them safe. There was a time when x-rays were considered safe for pregnant women. Ultrasounds have never conclusively been proven to be harmful, but they have also never conclusively been proven to be 100 per cent safe.

What If There's a Problem?

Although getting a scan is usually an exciting time for some parents, the news is not always good. If a problem shows up, make sure to ask the doctor or midwife the exact nature of the problem, how it might effect your baby, what your options are, etc.

Making the Best Choices for You and Your Baby

What About my Baby?

There has been a lot of focus on the mother's experience of birth and how different choices can affect her. What about the baby? How are our babies affected by the choices we make as expectant mothers?

Scientific research has shown how foetuses in the sixth month of pregnancy are aware and active and react to certain stimuli — both physical and emotional. Their senses are sufficiently developed that they can hear, smell and taste. (But before you start playing French tapes to your bump, at this point the only thing your baby needs to know is how much he is wanted.) Much research suggests that these experiences help the unborn child to learn about himself and his place in the world and can actually have a great effect on his personality development in later life. There have been significant advances in the study of how our babies are affected by our actions and feelings before and during birth. For example:

> In an interesting piece of research several years ago Dr Michael Lieberman showed that an unborn child grows emotionally agitated (measured by his heart rate) each time his mother *thinks* of having a cigarette. Just the idea of having a cigarette is enough to upset the baby. Of course, the baby has no way of knowing his mother is smoking or thinking about it but his brain is sophisticated enough to associate the experience of her smoking with the unpleasant sensation it produces in him. It puts him a constant state of uncertainty and fear. He just never knows when the unpleasant sensation will happen again. (*Source:* Thomas Verney and John Kelley, *The Secret Life of the Unborn Child*)

After months of floating peacefully, birth can be highly traumatic for your baby. **Oxytocin**, a hormone that our body produces in labour, has an amnesic affect (causes you to forget). It has been shown that birth memories can be retrieved with a qualified therapist. Dr David B. Cheek has, through hypnosis, been able to retrieve birth memories about specific incidents which only he would be aware of, such as the angle of the baby's head when it descends. If such details can be re- membered, what about those children who have traumatic births — emergency **caesarean section, forceps, vacuum**? How do these first experiences of life outside the womb affect their personalities? Similarly, how would a gentle birth experience affect him?

As mothers, all of our emotions are experienced by our babies. Although your baby doesn't yet have the vocabulary to understand what is being said around him, he feels stress when Mum is stressed and feels happy when Mum is happy. Isn't it time we put as much thought into our mental well-being as we do with our physical self?

TAKE A BABY BONDING BREAK TODAY!

You can send messages to your unborn child by the emotions you feel. The best way to send the message is by taking several baby breaks a day. First, find some music that you enjoy and that makes you feel good. Listen to music that gives you the feeling of peace, joy and love. It might be an old song that brings back happy memories or just the sound of the waves on the beach. (Get those endorphins going!) Play it so your unborn baby can hear it (don't use earphones) and then relax by taking several deep breaths while sitting or lying in a restful position. Fill your senses with a peaceful scene like a mountain lake or beach. Be sure to use all of your senses. See the ocean, hear the waves, feel the sand and sun, smell the salt air. This may take some practice, but after several attempts you will start feeling your own body's response to the mental picture. That's when you know you are sending a message to your baby.

I suggest you take a 20-minute baby bonding break once or twice a day — more if you're really feeling stressed. This practice has many benefits to you and to your unborn child. It will programme your child's emotional temperament and give him/her the expectation of peace and love in his or her universe after birth. Do it standing at the bus stop, or sitting in traffic — make it something easy to incorporate into what is no doubt an already busy life.

Many antenatal yoga classes include mother/baby bonding sessions, which is a wonderful way to get to know your baby before birth. We desperately need antenatal care that puts as much emphasis on the mother and child's emotional needs as it does on the physical ones.

Being aware of your unborn child's consciousness and awareness should make the birth planning process easier. When you understand that every choice you make can have a positive or negative effect on your baby, making the right decision gets a whole lot easier.

© Frederick Wirth MD. Adapted and reproduced with kind permission from Prenatal Parenting: The Complete Psychological and Spiritual Guide to Loving Your Unborn Child.

Each pregnancy and each birth is different. The following are two very different birth stories, the first of a number you will find in this book. (Please note that all names and some details of births have been changed, for all birth stories in this book.)

THERESE'S BIRTH STORY

My labour started on a Monday but at that stage I wasn't aware, as a first-time mum, that I was even in labour! I wasn't due for another two days; surely it couldn't be starting now! I had attended all of my antenatal classes, had got tips on what a Braxton Hicks was all about but still didn't know I was actually having a contraction on this Monday afternoon! I was bent over with pain and told myself that it was something I ate. I sat back down to watch TV and everything went back to normal.

On Tuesday morning I got up, had a shower and felt great. I went shopping and did all the normal things a girl does to prepare for the birth of her baby. I went crazy washing clothes that didn't need washing, dusted the house from top to bottom and cooked chicken that was already cooked! I went back to watching television, feet up . . . I felt just fine. Later that evening I felt completely exhausted and went to bed early about 8.00 pm. I kept wondering if I was going to deliver my baby on the expected due day, or would it be overdue by two weeks. I couldn't get comfortable and kept feeling a niggling pain all over my tummy. I was getting excited and thought "there's something going on"! I just couldn't relax and kept getting up to walk around.

I rang my sister Mary at about 10.00 pm to discuss it with her, as she had two children. She said this was the start of labour and I was even more excited. She told me to take a shower and time the contractions. At this stage they were coming every 30 minutes and bearable.

Mary said to stay at home until at least midnight and then she would collect me. I had already had a shower earlier that day and while having a second one my mother shouted up to me, "Why are you having another shower when you already had one this morning, you will wash yourself down the drain!" I didn't want to alarm her so I told her I was just trying to cool myself down. At about 11.20 pm Mary arrived; my mother asked what she was doing up at the house at that hour of the night. My sister replied "It's time!" That's when my mother started to panic!

At 11.30 pm the contractions were coming full force and I was doing my breathing techniques, which helped a great deal. We headed into the Rotunda Hospital and made it for 12.05 am. In the admissions room was told I was 5cm dilated and was asked if I wanted the epidural and I said "Yes!" We took the lift up to the delivery suite, where I met with my midwife who was lovely and so relaxed. I was so excited I couldn't wait to give birth. I already knew that my obstetrician was away for that bank holiday weekend, but surprised me by turning up just after I had given birth.

I got the epidural, which was scary to say the least. I didn't go for the gas or pethidine or anything else. It took over an hour to get the epidural needle, which quickly set in. When it did kick in, I felt great!

I was relaxed and the midwife asked me if I knew whether I was having a boy or a girl and I told her a girl as people had been telling me that I had "it all in the back and sides" and every time I went to a clothes shop for kids I was drawn to the pink section, so I had convinced myself that I was having a girl! I was chatting away when the midwife told me to start pushing; and push I did. A very short time later, at 3.30 am, I delivered a beautiful baby boy! I was very surprised but ecstatic when I realised it was a boy!

I have to say the whole experience of pregnancy and childbirth was surprising and enjoyable. I sailed through it. I was so absolutely overjoyed with the birth experience that I would have had another baby there and then! The staff were excellent and I even got a private room to share with my beautiful son alone! It was the happiest day of my life and I will treasure that for the rest of my life.

ANN'S BIRTH STORY

My son Jake was born at 10 am on a Saturday, three days before his due date. Being a first timer, I was quite idealistic about birth and certain I could cope with whatever came my way. I had read several books and attended both an active birth class and a regular antenatal class. Although I wanted to keep an open mind, I was hoping for a natural birth and made out a birth plan (amended several times) to reflect this.

It started off pretty well. A couple of days before the birth I felt very restless and had huge surges of energy. Everyone told me I would go overdue on my first, so I was surprised to feel a few funny little twinges on the Wednesday night. I thought they were kind of painful at the time (how naïve in

retrospect!) but decided I was constipated as I couldn't believe it was anything else.

By Thursday evening, they started feeling a little stronger. These were achy cramps in my belly that definitely didn't feel normal. I was excited and nervous but unwilling to think this could be labour on the way, as I had so expected to go overdue.

My husband Tony had just bought a car that week and was learning how to drive. We expected to have a few weeks so he could practise the route to the hospital. We went for a practice drive that evening but all the stopping and starting was increasing the pain. It was completely manageable, however, and we put it down to maybe strong Braxton-

Hicks. I had a glass of wine and a bath to relax me, but I was beginning to get pretty hyper now. I took advantage of this time and got plenty of massages and rolled around on my birthing ball.

In retrospect, I probably overdosed on active birth aids! I was hopping in and out of clary sage baths, trying various relaxation techniques, burning oils and pacing around the house all night. Needless to say, I was pretty exhausted by Friday morning. I hadn't slept and was starting to get very bored of amusing myself with aromatherapy and music while Tony slept soundly.

I had a "show" around 7.00 am and rang the hospital. The midwife on reception sounded quite blasé and told me to come in when contractions were three minutes apart. They were now about five to ten minutes apart but kept stopping and starting. I really wanted to wait at home as long as possible, so I went for a long walk with Tony, stopping every few minutes to bend into the contraction. It was all very weird and strangely enjoyable, just the two of us pretending to do normal things but with the anticipation of what lay ahead.

By nine that evening I felt I needed to get to the hospital. I'd had a bath and the pain really stepped up afterwards. I felt a bit sick and disorientated and was conscious of the shaky drive ahead. Tony got highly excited at my disorientated state and went to look it up in the books. "You're strange and confused. The books say you could be in transition!"

It couldn't be that quick, I thought. But the pain *was* very bad! We grabbed the bag and bundled into the car, convinced I was well on the way.

Neither of us will ever forget that drive. Tony's hands gripped the wheel until his knuckles were pure white. We drove through the city centre at 10.00 pm on a Friday, behind ambulances, police cars and pedestrians milling around. Tony missed the turn for the hospital three times and we went around in circles as he cursed and I kept quiet, breathing steadily through each pain.

We finally arrived in one piece. We were met by the midwife on duty. She berated me mildly for not coming in earlier and whisked me off to the examination room. Everything was done quickly and quietly. I think I may have been the only woman in labour there on a Friday night!

Tony was sent off to sign admittance forms and other documents that he admitted later to not really reading properly. I was swiftly hooked up to monitors and had an internal exam. I'd been dreading this but it was actually OK, not painful at all, just a little uncomfortable. I was convinced I would be well dilated; how disappointing to hear I was only 4 cm!

We were brought into a small little room with a bed, birthing ball and shower. It was dark and clinical and I suddenly felt really down and upset. Another long night stretched ahead and I didn't feel so in control anymore. Here in the hospital, I was just another woman in labour, to be dealt with quickly and professionally. All my breathing and labour techniques felt totally wrong here and I couldn't help wishing I'd stayed at home.

My consultant was away and had failed to deliver my birth plan to the midwives as he had promised. I had brought a copy with me and handed it over, a little shamefacedly I must admit.

The doctor on call took a look at my plan and said he fully supported my wish to birth without intervention. There was a proviso, however: I needed to get to 6 cm in the next three to four hours.

Talk about pressure! I was suddenly in a race, desperate to prove my competent cervix and superior labour ability to all these people. I thought with growing resentment of all those classes and books, describing contractions as "uncom-fortable" and pain as "positive"; friends with children hiding their mirth as I earnestly outlined my high pain threshold and desire for a natural birth.

But I still felt that I could do this and that Tony and I would manage on our own. I drank tea and ate toast, managing each contraction pretty well and chatting with Tony. In the back of my mind I was worried that time was going slowly. I was dying for something to happen.

After another internal, I was told I wasn't dilating. We discussed breaking my waters; I agreed as I wanted things to speed up. I felt it made sense but the pain was horrible. The procedure was quick but felt nasty and invasive. After that, the contractions came very fast.

I walked around, did some yoga and breathed through each contraction. Waves of immense pain were coming closer and now it was impossible to focus on anything else. I knew it was bad when I wasn't able to drink juice or touch any of my high glucose snacks. I didn't want to be on all fours, on the birthing ball or have Tony near me.

Massages didn't work any more and I was getting desperate to find something to distract me. Part of me wished to be offered pain relief but I'd asked not to be offered it in my birth plan and was too stubborn to request it! However, I still felt I could just about control the pain by greeting it and breathing into it. I sat on the floor for ages and just meditated as best I could. I remember visualising the contractions: sometimes they were waves of white light building up from the pelvis right through my insides; sometimes I was climbing a hill and peaking and descending. It was all so long, sickening and exhausting.

I didn't move or disturb the rhythm as the midwife and Tony sat silently with me and watched. I was determined not to cry or groan as I feared that I would descend into panic if I did. I was so quiet that the midwife told me it was hard to believe a woman was in labour. She tried to encourage me but I really needed a new diversion now, something else to help me.

I was monitored and examined again and getting pretty impatient with all these procedures! The internal showed I had only moved 1 cm in the last few hours. I was 5 cm and completely demoralised.

The baby's heartbeat wasn't picking up too well anymore on the monitor. The doctor came in and examined me. He said the baby's head seemed quite small and that he was in the posterior position. He was worried about the heartbeat and, although he

understood I didn't want a C-section, it might be necessary. I was getting close to not caring by then. I was knackered and nauseous. I couldn't even drink water and I was really scared of the pain getting even worse — which the doctor assured me it would.

I took a shower and the hot water helped a little but I was getting confused and angry. I wanted someone to tell me what to do, or just to tell me I could do this, that I was managing. I had lost faith in my ability to do this. I was terrified and I wanted to go home!

The heart rate was still not picking up too well after contractions. The doctor suggested putting in a syntocinon drip to speed things up. He added that I'd find this very painful and would need an epidural as the contractions would be a lot worse. He added that a C-section was looking more and more likely if we didn't move fast to speed things up. I still felt I might manage it but I didn't know how much longer they would let me go on without a dreaded C-section. Plus the prospect of pain relief suddenly sounded like heaven.

Another hour passed before the anaesthetist arrived. I hadn't realised how high on natural endorphins I was until they hooked me up and turned on the drugs. As pain relief gradually flooded my body I felt all the adrenaline leave with a "whoosh".

All the voices and images in my head left suddenly and I lay on the delivery table, being turned and prodded, hooked up to all sorts of monitors, feeling a mixture of relief, shame and depression.

Having no pain was amazing and the awful fatigue and sickness left my body. But I felt I could have kept going, that I had "given in" somehow. I was also lost without my need to breathe and meditate. Tony went off for breakfast and I was alone with a new midwife on duty and an uninterested doctor. I lay there feeling sorry for myself, refusing to sleep.

As it turned out, I only had to wait an hour in that state. I was checked again and the syntocinon drip had worked its magic — I was 7 cm by now.

But the baby's heart rate was dropping and not recovering very well. The doctor told me again that a C-section might be necessary but we'd "try some pushing" first . . .

All this happened so fast. Tony said later he came back from breakfast and there I was on the table, legs akimbo and held up by midwives, starting to push. I delivered myself into their hands. This was the real deal — when it really happens. I don't think I can ever remember living so intensely in the moment as when I pushed. I visualised the rectum and held my breath as I bore down and used every ounce of my strength.

And they cheered me on, told me I was doing great — all the things I had dreaded. Even worse, I found myself somehow with my legs in stirrups — exactly what I had set out to avoid. I had pictured myself elegantly squatting and delivering the baby with a few quick pushes!

But it didn't matter right now. I was too caught up really participating again, now more than ever — and I liked it once I understood what I was doing. I breathed and pushed with incredible strength for 30 minutes and my son slithered out with one last almighty push.

And then this tiny, scared little creature plopped onto my tummy. His eyes were wide open and he looked straight up at me. I looked at him in astonishment and everything else ceased to exist for a moment.

I'm sure I cried but it's all a bit of a blur after that. I was unable to grasp it was all over and he was here. The team around me moved with ruthless efficiency, cleaning up the mess; the doctor chatted away as he gave me some stitches and Jake was whisked off to be put in an incubator as he was so small — only 4lbs 10oz.

I was given some tea and toast which tasted amazing and Tony and I were left alone for a while. We could hardly string words together; we were both shell shocked. I felt wired but also pretty confused. I wanted to relive every moment of the birth again and again and talk about every detail.

Jake was kept in the Special Care Unit for a week. In the days that followed I discovered that my placenta had most likely stopped functioning, which explained why he was so small. He had shown up as about 6lb on the last scan two weeks before the birth, so had most likely lost weight in the womb. I never found out for sure what happened or whether it could have been avoided.

I can't say that birth was a joyous experience for me; the whole experience was overwhelming and it took me a while to get over it. While I am glad that I did arm myself with knowledge and a good birth plan, I know now that these can only take you so far. It's hard not to be a little idealistic your first time round and wish for a wonderful labour. My labour may not have been easy, but it had its wonderful moments!

EVIDENCE-BASED CARE

There's a new catchphrase in medicine: "**evidence-based care**". Evidence-based maternity care involves using the best research about the safety and effectiveness of specific tests, treatments and other interventions to help guide maternity care decisions. In a nutshell, evidence-based medicine is care based on the recommendations of the highest quality research available. To take a simple example, outside the area of maternity: suppose your sister falls and twists her ankle badly. Her doctor would follow guidelines specific to your sister's situation: after an examination, if all the signs point to there being a break, he would recommend an x-ray. Clinical recommendations drawn up following randomised controlled studies (the gold standard of research) show that the best course of action in this case is to confirm that there is a broken bone by taking an x-ray. This would be the practice of evidence-based medicine. Of course, the doctor could also have just sent your sister home with a set of crutches and a pressure bandage and told her to stay off her foot for a few days because, in his opinion, there are no bones broken. This would not be evidence-based medicine.

All maternity care needs to reflect "best practice" principles and be evidence-based. Telling you that your shoe size or your height will affect your chances of a successful vaginal birth would not be evidence-based care. Unfortunately, it seems that obstetrics takes a lot longer to follow evidence-based practices than most other areas of medicine. A good example of non-evidence-based policies often seen in Irish hospitals is the restriction of food and water to labouring mothers — more on this later.

The following piece sheds some international light on how Ireland's maternity system has developed. The author, Marsden Wagner, MD, is a perinatologist and perinatal epidemiologist from California and an outspoken supporter of midwifery. He was director of Women's and Children's Health in the World Health Organisation for 15 years.

FISH CAN'T SEE WATER

By Marsden Wagner

Humanising birth means understanding that the woman giving birth is a human being, not a machine and not just a container for making babies. Showing women — half of all people — that they are inferior and inadequate by taking away their power to give birth is a tragedy for all society. On the other hand, respecting the woman as an important and valuable human being and making certain that the woman's experience while giving birth is fulfilling and empowering is not just a nice extra; it is absolutely essential as it makes the woman strong and therefore makes society strong.

But we do not have humanised birth in many places today. Why? Because fish can't see the water they swim in. Birth attendants, be they doctors, midwives or nurses, who have experienced only hospital-based, high interventionist, medicalised birth cannot see the profound effect their interventions are having on the birth.

These hospital birth attendants have no idea what a birth looks like without all the interventions, a birth which is not dehumanised. This widespread inability to know what normal, humanised birth is has been summarised by the WHO:

"By medicalising birth, i.e. separating a woman from her own environment and surrounding her with strange people using strange machines to do strange things to her in an effort to assist her, the woman's state of mind and body is so altered that her way of carrying through this intimate act must also be altered and the state of the baby born must equally be altered. The result is that it is no longer possible to know what births would have been like before these manipulations. Most health care providers no longer know what 'non-medicalised' birth is. The entire modern obstetric and neonatological literature is essentially based on observations of 'medicalised' birth." (World Health Organisation).

Why is medicalised birth necessarily dehumanising? In medicalised birth the doctor is always in control while the key element in humanised birth is the woman in control of her own birthing and whatever happens to her.

There is an expectation that there are guarantees of perfect outcomes with childbirth. **Obstetricians** are trained to think that "doing something is better than doing nothing" since the introduction of a high-tech approach to birth. It has lulled women and health professionals alike into a false sense of security that by providing the very best of appropriate care we can always avoid an unexpected outcome.

Although obstetric care is slowly becoming more evidence-based, there is a tendency not to evaluate routine interventions for their subtle and/or long-term risks. Another reason for the gap between evidence and practice is the excuses often given by consultants for why they reject evidence in their medical practice. These excuses include: the evidence is out of date; collecting evidence is too slow and prevents progress; they use clinical judgement and their opinion and experience; using anecdotal "horror stories" to try to prove the need for an intervention which the evidence has found unnecessary; quoting evidence which is of poor and/or inadequate quality; "trust me, I am a doctor".

In addition to these excuses, in maternity care common excuses include: our women have smaller pelvises (no evidence). Obstetricians tend to blind faith in technology and the mantra: technology = progress = modern. The other side of the coin is the lack of faith in nature, best expressed by a Canadian obstetrician: "Nature is a bad obstetrician."

Doctors replaced midwives for low-risk births, then science proved midwives safer. Hospital replaced home for low-risk birth, then science proved home as safe with far less unnecessary intervention. Hospital staff replaced family as birth support, then science proved birth safer if family present. Lying on your back replaced vertical birth positions, and then science proved vertical positions safer. Newborn examinations away from mothers in the first 20 minutes replaced leaving babies with mothers, then science proved the necessity for maternal attachment during this time. Man-made milk replaced woman-made milk, then science proved breastmilk superior. The central nursery replaced the mother, then science proved rooming-in superior. The incubator replaced the mother's body for care of low-weight newborns, then science proved the kangaroo method better in many cases.

© *Marsden Wagner. Adapted and reproduced with kind permission.*

So what does all this mean to you? Well, if your consultant or midwife *routinely* does **episiotomies**; recommends withholding food during labour; insists that you birth on the bed; automatically recommends c-section for a **breech, posterior** or even just a big baby without offering other options . . . they are not practising evidence-based care. You can choose to stay with this consultant or find one that shares the same philosophy on birth as you do.

The following article from a great resource, MaternityWise.org (The Maternity Center Association) explains the importance of making informed choices in your care.

INFORMED DECISION MAKING, INFORMED CONSENT AND INFORMED REFUSAL

By the Maternity Center Association

You are responsible for making informed decisions, and you have the legal right to give "informed consent" or "informed refusal".

Why is my involvement in maternity care decisions important?

As a pregnant woman, you have the opportunity and responsibility to make many important decisions about your care during pregnancy, birth and the time after birth. The decisions you make and the maternity care you receive can have lasting effects on the health and well-being of your baby, yourself and your family.

It is always important to understand whether there is a good rationale for any procedure, drug, test or treatment that is being given or offered to you. In many care settings, certain practices are used freely and even routinely, whether or not the mother or baby has shown a clear need. Although these practices may be of value to women or babies in certain situations, they may be unnecessary for most. They may be disruptive, be uncomfortable, cause more serious side effects and lead to the use of other interventions. For these reasons, interventions should not be used routinely or unnecessarily.

What does "making informed decisions" about maternity care mean?

Making informed decisions means learning and thinking about the best information available on maternity care, and then deciding what's right for you. Key questions for you to consider are:

- What are the possible choices?

- What does the best available research tell us about the safety and effectiveness of each of these choices?

- What are my needs and preferences and those of other family members?

- What choices are available and supported in my care setting?

- If I want an option that will not or may not be available to me, would I consider switching to a care setting or caregiver that does offer my preferred care?

Whenever possible, it's important to weigh this information well before you need to decide. This will ensure that you can get answers to all of your questions and have access to the kind of care that is right for you.

How can I find the best evidence about safe and effective maternity care?

Dedicated health professionals also struggle to keep up with the vast amount of information relating to their practice and to know how to provide the best care.

Archie Cochrane, originator of the Cochrane Collaboration (a wonderful tool for researching evidence-based medicine) wondered which bits of medicine deserved the gold medal for being the most scientifically based and which deserved the wooden spoon for being the least scientific. . . . eventually he decided that it was the obstetricians that deserved the wooden spoon for being the least scientific doctors on the planet.

Fortunately, the evidence-based health care movement can help consumers and professionals alike sort out these complex matters.

What can I do to help ensure that the care that I receive during labour and birth will be best for me and my baby?

Your choice of caregiver and choice of birth setting (home or hospital) can have a major impact on the care that you receive during labour and birth. You may need to explore many possibilities to find a caregiver and birth setting that offer care consistent with the best evidence and with your needs and preferences.

It's not possible to know ahead of time exactly what your birth experience will be like. Being as informed as possible in advance will help you deal wisely with any new decisions that may arise at the time. It is important to learn about your options, get answers to your questions and think about your preferences well before labour begins. Be sure your partner, if you have one, is also aware of your wishes and is prepared to speak on your behalf if the need arises.

What does it mean to give "informed consent"?

Informed consent is a process to help you decide what will and will not be done to you and your body. In the case of maternity care, informed consent also gives you the authority to decide about care that affects your baby. The purpose of informed consent is to respect your right to self-determination. It empowers you with the authority to decide what options are in the best interest of you and your baby. Your rights to autonomy, to the truth (as best as it can be known at the time), and to keep yourself and your children safe and free of harm are very basic human rights.

What are my legal rights to "Informed Consent" and "Informed Refusal"?

Whenever a medical procedure, drug, test or other treatment is offered to you, you have the legal right to "informed consent". This means that your doctor, midwife or nurse is responsible for explaining:

- Why this type of care is being offered

- What it would involve

- The risks and benefits that are associated with this type of care

- Alternatives to this care, and their respective risks and benefits, including doing nothing (that is, simply waiting longer).

You have a right to clear and full explanations about your care. You are entitled to get answers to any and all questions that you may have about your care. You are also within your rights to request and receive a copy of your medical records and to get a second opinion.

Then, by law, you have the right to decide whether to accept the care that is offered. If you disagree with your caregiver and decide not to accept care that is offered to you, this is called "informed refusal". And, even if you have made your decision and signed a form agreeing to a particular type of care, you have the right to change your mind.

It can be challenging to carry out the informed consent process in the context of busy health care routines. Yet, you and your caregiver can set aside the time to discuss these issues in advance whenever possible and again when it is time to make a decision. You don't want to be learning about procedures and options for the first time when you're in labour and facing important decisions.

What are some tips for exploring these issues with my doctor or midwife?

Make a list of your questions before each visit, and take notes on the answers. You may wish to bring your partner or someone else close to you along to listen to what is said. Don't be shy; nothing is off-limits. While talking with your caregiver, don't hesitate to say:

- I don't understand.

- Please explain this to me.

- What could happen to me or my baby if I do that? Or if I don't?

- What are my other options?

- Where can I get more information about what you're recommending?

- I have some information I'd like to share with you.

- I'm uncomfortable with what you are recommending.

- I'm not ready to make a decision yet.

- I'm thinking about getting a second opinion.

And remember, any question that you have is a question worth asking. It's important to let your caregiver know when you don't understand. Ask again, until you do.

What happens if my caregiver and I disagree?

Your caregiver has rights, too. He or she has the right to agree or disagree to provide care that you may request. For example, if you request a caesarean and have no medical need for this procedure, your caregiver has the right to refuse to do the surgery.

Use your BRAIN to help you make informed choices

- **B** — what are the **Benefits** of this (test, intervention, etc.)?
- **R** — what are the **Risks** associated with this course of action?
- **A** — what are my **Alternatives**?
- **I** — what is my **Intuition** telling me?
- **N** — what if we do **Nothing** or just wait a while?

HOW TO CHOOSE YOUR CAREGIVER

Many Western doctors hold the belief that we can improve everything, even natural childbirth in a healthy woman. This philosophy is the philosophy of people who think it deplorable that they were not consulted at the creation of Eve, because they would have done a better job. (Kloosterman, 1994)

We spend more time finding a good travel agent than we do, as mothers-to-be, finding the right caregiver to guide us through pregnancy and birth. Birth planning can determine if your current doctor/ midwife is the best match for you. But how can you find this out? If you are a private patient then it's easy — you just ask a few creatively worded questions. If you don't like the response you get, then you interview another doctor until you find one who is on the same page as you are. If you are a semi-private patient, your choices aren't as good. You'll meet a team of doctors and you have no idea who will show up on the big day, but you can still ask the questions. For public patients the options aren't much better because again you won't know who will be caring for you during your labour.

Obstetrician-Led Care Versus Midwife-Led Care

When you are deciding where to have your baby, you'll probably be choosing from different places and options such as:

- Midwife-led unit: Currently only available in Drogheda or Cavan (for public patients only)

- Hospital: Obstetrician

- Hospital: Community midwives (for public patients only)

- Home birth service.

Obstetricians are trained in abnormal and complicated births. According to the World Health Organisation:

> Generally obstetricians have to devote their attention to high-risk women and the treatment of serious complications. They are normally responsible for obstetric surgery. By training and by professional attitude they may be inclined and indeed, are often required by the situation, to intervene more frequently than the midwife. In many countries, especially in the developing world, the number of obstetricians is limited and they are unequally distributed, with the majority practising in big cities. Their responsibilities for the management of major complications are unlikely to leave them much time to assist and support the woman and her family for the duration of normal labour and delivery. Obstetricians in many countries have concluded that care during normal childbirth should be similar to the care in complicated deliveries. This concept has several disadvantages: it has the potential to turn a normal physiological event into a medical procedure; it interferes with the freedom of women to experience the birth of their children in their own way, in the place of their own choice; it leads to unnecessary interventions; and, because of the need for economies of scale, its application requires a concentration of large numbers of labouring women in technically well-equipped hospitals with the concomitant costs. Staff in referral facilities can become dysfunctional if their capacity to care for very sick

women who need all their attention and expertise is swamped by the sheer number of normal births which present themselves. In their turn, such normal births are frequently managed with "standardised protocols" which only find their justification in the care of women with childbirth complications.

Midwives are trained in normal birth (about 80 per cent of all births). In an ideal world, you would never see a consultant (obstetrician) unless you had a problem in your pregnancy. All of your prenatal care would be undertaken by midwives. Seeing an obstetrician for a normal pregnancy is like taking a two-year-old to a specialist paediatrician any time he gets a cold.

All current research supports midwife-led care for low-risk pregnancies — the vast majority of pregnancies in Ireland. Unfortunately, maternity care is mostly obstetrician-led in Ireland. Fear forms a huge part of what is driving the current model of managed obstetric care. If we were not so terrified of our bodies and pregnancy from childhood— a terror bred through the ignorance of society, culture and medicine — then it would make absolute sense for women to automatically choose a midwife when they become pregnant.

Similarly, there are essentially two very different ways of caring for a pregnant woman: **active management** (obstetrician-led) and **expectant management** (midwife-led). Many obstetricians and some hospital midwives see birth as a medical emergency, one that needs to be monitored continuously. In some hospitals in Ireland, this is tied to the notion that the success of your birth is purely dependent on whether you have efficient or inefficient **contractions**. Active management takes away the personal care that pregnant women need and reduces them to the numbers of contractions plotted on a chart. This is what's also known as the "production line" model of care.

According to the active management philosophy a woman's labour is only considered "normal" if she gives birth within the hospital's time limits — usually twelve hours. If you do not dilate according to the active management guidelines, you can expect to be encouraged to have your labour speeded up with artificial hormones. Which is fine if you've got someplace you need to be . . . However, most women don't like to be rushed when we're doing something important, such as giving birth.

Expectant management care is generally practised by most community and independent midwives and a few consultants who see pregnancy and birth as a significant but normal part of a woman's life and have more of a "wait and see" attitude. A consultant or midwife with an expectant management approach will encourage you to be actively involved in your own care and to be fully engaged in all decision-making, will encourage birth plans and will expect you to ask questions. Caregivers with this philosophy will not routinely schedule **inductions** or break your waters. Expectant management means your labour is viewed as natural, unless there are medical signs that suggest otherwise, and that your body knows what to do. Your care provider follows your lead with no, or very little, intervention. On the other hand, an active management caregiver takes the active role and manages your labour through intervention.

Of course, it is not simply a matter of asking your consultant or midwife if they practise active management or expectant management. Some caregivers (and hospitals) may have very medicalised (active management) policies on certain issues, such as determining when they feel an episiotomy is necessary, while they may have a more expectant management philosophy on, say, whether or not to speed up or augment labour.

So, there are many points in between the "extremes" of active and expectant management. Only you can decide at what point you would feel most comfortable, and try to find a caregiver who is sympathetic to your needs. Read up (in this book and elsewhere) and become informed about inductions, caesareans, episiotomies, etc., and ask your caregiver relevant questions about their policies. If you are not happy that they are meeting your expectations, it *is* possible to change to a different caregiver. Of course, this is not easy to do when you're a public patient, which is why having a birth plan (see pages 54–57) is so important — on the big day, you won't know who will be there to help you birth your baby. If you're a private patient and seeing a consultant that isn't working out, don't try to get your consultant to change — change consultant! Talk to women who have had the kinds of birth you want and find out who their consultant was.

CHOOSING A HOSPITAL

Established in the US in 1996, the Coalition for Improving Maternity Services (CIMS) is a collaborative effort of numerous individuals and more than 50 organisations representing over 90,000 members. Their mission is to promote a "wellness model" of maternity care that will improve birth outcomes and substantially reduce costs.

A group of experts in birthing care came up with a list of ten things to look for and ask about. Medical research supports all of these things. These are also the best ways to be mother-friendly. Here's what you should expect, and ask for, in your birth experience. Be sure to find out how the people you talk with handle these ten issues about caring for you and your baby:

TEN QUESTIONS TO ASK YOUR HOSPITAL

1. Who can be with me during labour and birth?

Mother-friendly, midwife-led units, hospitals and home birth services will let a birthing mother decide whom she wants to have with her during the birth. This includes fathers, partners, children, other family members or friends (and should not be restricted to just one birth partner).

They will also let a birthing mother have with her a person who has special training in helping women cope with labour and birth. This person is called a doula or labour support person. She never leaves the birthing mother alone. She encourages her, comforts her and helps her understand what's happening to her.

They will have midwives as part of their staff so that a birthing mother can have a midwife with her if she wants to. The WHO is supportive of women having a choice in their birth supporters.

---

2. What happens during a normal labour and birth in your setting?

If they give mother-friendly care, they will tell you how they handle every part of the birthing process. For example, how often do they give the mother a drug to speed up the birth? Or do they let labour and birth usually happen on its own timing?

They will also tell you how often they do certain procedures. For example, they will have a record of the percentage of C-sections they do every year. If the number is too high, you'll want to consider having your baby in another place or with another doctor or midwife.

Here are some numbers CIMS recommend you ask about:

- They should *not* try to start labour for more than one in ten women (10%) (the average in Ireland is about 25%).

- They should not do an episiotomy on more than one in five women (20%) (the average in Ireland is 25%). They should be trying to bring that number down.

- They should not do C-sections on more than one in ten women (10%) if it's a public hospital. The rate should be 15% or less in hospitals which care for many high-risk mothers and babies. (Sadly Ireland has one of the highest rates of caesareans in Europe at 25%).

- Mothers who have had a C-section can often have future babies vaginally (**VBAC**). Look for a birthplace in which six out of ten women (60%) or more of the mothers who have had C-sections go on to have VBAC for later births.

3. How do you allow for differences in culture and beliefs?

Mother-friendly birth centres, hospitals, and home birth services are sensitive to the mother's culture. They know that mothers and families have differing beliefs, values and customs.

For example, you may have a custom that only women may be with you during labour and birth. Or perhaps your beliefs include a religious ritual to be performed after birth. There are many other examples that may be very important to you. If the place and the people are mother-friendly, they will support you in doing what you want to do. Before labour starts, tell your doctor or midwife special things you want.

4. Can I walk and move around during labour? What position do you suggest for birth?

In mother-friendly settings, you can walk around and move about as you choose during labour. You can choose the positions that are most comfortable and work best for you during labour and birth. (There may be a medical reason for you to be in a certain position.) Mother-friendly settings almost never put a woman flat on her back for birth.

5. How do you make sure everything goes smoothly when my nurse, doctor, midwife or agency need to work with each other? Can my midwife come with me if I have to be moved to another place during labour?

Mother-friendly places and people will have a specific plan for keeping in touch with the other people who are caring for you. They will talk to others who give you birth care. They will help you find people or agencies in your community to help you. For example, they may put you in touch with someone who can help you with breastfeeding.

6. What things do you normally do to a woman in labour?

Experts say some methods of care during labour and birth are better and healthier for mothers and babies. Medical research shows us which methods of care are better and healthier. Mother-friendly settings only use methods that have been proven to be best by scientific evidence.

Here is a list of things we recommend you ask about. They do not help and may hurt healthy mothers and babies. They are not proven to be best for the mother or baby and are not mother-friendly:

- They should not keep track of the baby's heart rate all the time with a machine (called an electronic foetal monitor). Instead it is best to have your nurse or midwife listen to the baby's heart from time to time.

- They should not routinely break your bag of waters early in labour.

- They should not use an IV (a needle put into your vein to give you fluids).

- They should not tell you that you can't eat or drink during labour.

A birth centre, hospital or home birth service that does these things for most of the mothers is not mother-friendly. Remember, these should not be used without a special medical reason.

7. How do you help mothers stay as comfortable as they can be? Besides drugs, how do you help mothers relieve the pain of labour?

The people who care for you should know how to help you cope with labour. They should know about ways of dealing with your pain that don't use drugs — this is true midwifery care. They should suggest such things as changing your position, relaxing in a warm bath, having a massage and using music. These are called comfort measures.

Comfort measures help you handle your labour more easily and help you feel more in control. The people who care for you will not try to persuade you to use a drug for pain unless you need it to take care of a special medical problem. All drugs affect the baby.

8. What if my baby is born early or has special problems?

Mother-friendly places and people will encourage mothers and families to touch, hold, breastfeed and care for their babies as much as they can. They will encourage this even if your baby is born early or has a medical problem at birth. (However, there may be a special medical reason you shouldn't hold and care for your baby.)

9. Do you circumcise baby boys?

Medical research does not show a need to circumcise baby boys. It is painful and risky. Mother-friendly birth places discourage circumcision unless it is for religious reasons. Fortunately this is not an issue in Ireland yet.

10. How do you help mothers who want to breastfeed?

The World Health Organisation made this list of ways birth services support breastfeeding:

- They tell all pregnant mothers why and how to breastfeed.

- They help you start breastfeeding within one hour after your baby is born.

- They show you how to breastfeed. And they show you how to keep your milk coming in even if you have to be away from your baby for work or other reasons.

- Newborns should have only breastmilk. (However, there may be a medical reason they cannot have it right away.)

- They encourage you and the baby to stay together all day and all night. This is called "rooming-in".

- They encourage you to feed your baby whenever he or she wants to nurse, rather than at certain times.

- They should not give pacifiers ("dummies" or "soothers") to breastfed babies.

- They encourage you to join a group of mothers who breastfeed. They tell you how to contact a group near you.

- They have a written policy on breastfeeding. All the employees know about and use the ideas in the policy.

- They teach employees the skills they need to carry out these steps.

© *Coalition for the Improvement of Maternity Services (CIMS).*
www.motherfriendly.org

GRAINNE'S FIRST BIRTH EXPERIENCE

The birth of my first baby took place at the beginning of last year in an Irish hospital. Following a routine visit, on a Wednesday, to my consultant (a stand-in, as mine was on holidays) from the scan she said she could see a decrease in the amount of fluid and was sending me in to be induced. She asked if I noticed a reduction in movements. I said yes but that I felt it was due to the baby growing, and that I still had movement. However, she said that, based on this information and on her findings from the scan, I should be induced that night. Not knowing any different at that time, I agreed.

That night the consultant was too busy and I was told it would take place in the morning. All day Thursday I was monitored and the baby traced. Again I think the delay was because they were too busy. I was even allowed into town to go shopping and told to come back to the hospital later that evening!

I was finally induced on Friday afternoon. It was never explained to me what this entailed, the effects on me or my baby or what I should expect. The first attempt was not happening quickly enough for their liking so I was given an-

other half dose a while later. Following this, about 5.00 pm, the contractions came hard and fast. I requested the epidural as I was terrified. I was told I could go for it shortly. I had read that to be mobile helps, so I walked up and down corridors but I was in agony. I was then told by a midwife that a more urgent case had taken priority and I must wait a little longer for the epidural. I continued walking around for another few hours until I couldn't go on anymore and again asked about the epi. I was again told, "Sorry, but someone else has turned up and needed the delivery room so it'll be another while before we've a room free".

I continued alone and I was dilating ever so slowly but the pain was severe (as I found out later, induction makes the pain much more intense). Seven hours after I first asked about the epi, I called a midwife to find out what the situation was. She said she'd find out and a third time returned to tell me, "Sorry, but we're really busy tonight and someone else needed the delivery room again". She then said she could give me an injection of pethidine for the pain. I was in agony and agreed and so it was administered. Again, what this meant was not explained, nor were the effects mentioned. I only later found out about the risks to the unborn baby.

At 7.00 am the following morning I was eventually brought to the delivery section, but not to a suite, just to where I could use gas and air. I remained there for another few hours until a room came free. On examination by a registrar there, I overheard him say to a colleague, "She never had decreased waters." He left the room and I didn't see him again to pursue this, though I wasn't in the frame of mind to pursue it anyway. But of course if this *was* true I presume I would never have needed to be induced!

I was eventually brought into the delivery suite. Not long after I felt the need to push, and asked the midwife what to do. I was told to just push when I had a contraction so I remember trying to fight against pushes and it felt awful. She would also disappear out of the room for short periods, leaving just me and my husband. I had to get him to call the midwife when I thought I should push, as I wanted to make sure I was doing it properly. It was chaotic.

My recollection of the rest is still traumatic for me. After an endless time of pushing, where I felt my heart was going to explode (my husband later told me my face was as purple as could be; he thought I would burst), I told the midwife I didn't feel I could go on. I was so tired, had no energy left, was in horrendous pain and was starting to feel like a failure. The midwife told me she'd get the consultant.

So a male consultant appeared, examined me and then told me he'd be back to give me some help! When he returned he was armed with instruments and when he opened them out I nearly had a stroke. He then performed an episiotomy, without explanation or my consent, and proceeded to insert a vacuum, again without explanation/consent.

He asked me to tell him when I had a contraction. When I said one was coming the midwife shook her head as if to indicate I was wrong; the consultant asked the midwife "does she?" How demeaning! I definitely felt at this point as though I didn't have a clue, as I was even being told when I was or wasn't having a contraction, like I didn't know my own body! I insisted I had a contraction coming and the midwife said, "Well, I suppose she'd feel them first."

Eventually it ended and my beautiful baby girl was put on my chest for a moment. Although I say that now, at the time I was in such shock from this horrendous experience that I didn't even take it in. I was wheeled back to my room carrying my baby; I barely remember the journey I was so traumatised.

I now well up even recalling all of this. I feel that what should have been the most exciting and memorable time of my life was robbed from me by this despicable hospital experience.

I am now both saddened by it but also very angry. A short time ago I expressed my dissatisfaction in a letter to the hospital administrator. The response was that an investigation would take place; and the outcome of that was an apology, but not from anyone in particular. So I don't actually know who is sorry, but I know it's worded that way so no one is held accountable for legal reasons. Also, everything I described here was justified in his responding letter. So, with no real remorse from them I must just let it lie but am still very bitter and very afraid of ever becoming pregnant again. I obviously love my baby immensely and am delighted she is here.

LOUISE'S BIRTH STORY

My name is Louise and I would like to tell my "birth story". I am 29 and was due my second baby in March 2005. It was our older son's seventh birthday that day and he was really looking forward to his big birthday present. His birthday came and there was no sign of this little one coming. As I had my antenatal check-up that day my doctor asked me should he stretch the membranes a little. I was delighted as this had worked wonders on James and had started labour that time. And it worked again, albeit a little slower this time. I had very light contractions all night and couldn't sleep in anticipation of what would happen. I finally got up at seven o'clock in the morning and was disappointed as my contractions were still only very light and came only every 15 minutes. There was no way I was going to wait another day — this baby was coming out today and that was that!

So myself, my partner Conor and James all went for a long walk, then I took a bath and then went for another walk. At around 4.00 pm we dropped Max off at his granny's house and made our way to the hospital. There I walked some more. At 7.30 pm — after about six hours of walking — I was admitted. Conor went home for a while and I walked some more!

Finally at 11.30 pm, my waters broke. However, my contractions, although quite strong, were still very short, which meant my cervix was only dilating quite slowly. I went back up to the delivery room and was told . . . yes, to walk some more. Conor was massaging my back as I walked the corridors of the hospital, I can still see them in front of me!

By 1.00 am I had had enough. I was exhausted so I asked the nurse for the epidural. As I was 3 cm dilated at this stage the nurse agreed. However, while we waited for the anaesthetist, the baby's heart rate started to increase. This worried the doctor increasingly and we were told they would have to take blood from the baby's head. At this stage I was on gas and air but the contractions were about 45 seconds long and came every minute and a half. Conor had to leave the room and I can only imagine how worried he must have been for the next 15 minutes. They were the longest 15 minutes of my life! I knew deep down that there would be no time for the epidural, the contractions were too painful and too long and I already felt like pushing towards the end.

When the results came back from the lab the doctor was happy enough to give me the epidural, but after examining me he found I was 8 cm dilated so there was no time. I cried! I could not imagine going through this pain for the next hour. I needn't have worried: the second stage of my labour lasted only three minutes and after pushing three times, our beautiful baby girl was born at 3.18 am.

The cord was wrapped around her neck quite tightly and that was the reason she had been so distressed. She had also pooped in the womb just prior to birth, which again was an indication of how distressed she had been. She was put on my lap and I could not believe how similar she looked to her older brother — they were identical! I was in a daze, but looking at her I knew there was something wrong. Instead of breathing she was grunting and she was a bluish colour. I immediately panicked and kept saying: "She's not breathing, she's not breathing!" They examined her and gave her oxygen, but it took minutes until she stopped grunting. They then told us she would have to go to the ICU for a little while. Their information was very sketchy but they reassured us it was because she had been born too quickly and was nothing to worry about.

It is difficult to describe the feeling in that delivery room. The room was so empty and we had so many questions. Was she OK? Why did they rush her off? Was there something they were not telling us? Did she have brain damage? I think that was the biggie. Neither of us wanted to ask that question. We wouldn't have been ready for the answer. In what seemed like an eternity I got showered and dressed in my pyjamas and then we sat there waiting to be taken to ICU.

We finally went to see her at around 6.00 am. She was in an incubator with tubes everywhere and her eyes were wide open. She was looking at me, sucking on her fingers. I kept thinking, she's only so small, she can't understand why I'm not with her. I will never forget this incredible feeling of helplessness and this urge to just hold her. The doctors told us she had a pneumothorax, a collapsed lung and therefore she needed oxygen. The oxygen would help to reduce the air bubble which had escaped her lung into the chest. It was apparently very small so it wasn't too serious. It would take a day or two to clear. As there had been meconium in the womb they also wanted to give her antibiotics to avoid a possible infection.

There it was. It didn't sound all that serious but part of us was convinced they were trying to protect us and weren't telling us everything. There was nothing we could do. I had to leave my beautiful new baby "on her own" and go downstairs to my bed. I had such mixed feelings; I didn't know if she was going to be OK . . . Could she die? Was there permanent damage? . . .

She was on oxygen for two days and I was not allowed to take her into my arms for those two days. I couldn't even take her out to feed her. I had to express milk and they had to feed her through a tube into her nose. It was very hard to sit in the ward looking at the other new mums with their new babies and mine wasn't there. I cannot describe the joy I felt when I could finally take her down to the ward with me on the third day of her life. Finally she was there beside me and she was OK.

Isabel is now nearly six months old and she is the happiest baby ever! She has never been sick and the doctors have reassured us that there will be no lasting effects on her health. Although it was definitely not the labour of my dreams, she makes up for that a hundred times over!

Choosing Your Birth Partner

Your bag is packed. You've finally figured out the car seat and your partner has just finished assembling the cot with *Krypton Factor*-like precision. Your guess date is fast approaching. It's time to think about who can best support you during the exciting — and sometimes scary — hours of labour. Just as you carefully selected your consultant or midwife, your choice of birth partner is an important decision.

I'm sure you are aware of the old Hollywood cliché of the anxious expectant father pacing the corridors of the hospital, waiting for good news; his first glimpse of his new baby only coming when some smiling nurse holds the infant up to him from a glassed-in nursery. This was followed by the celebratory cigar. Thankfully, those days are long gone (if they ever really existed) and hospitals welcome birth partners, whether they are husbands, mothers, sisters, friends or even a doula (professional labour supporter). If you're having a doula you'll need to get permission from the head of obstetrics.

Mothers, sisters or friends who have already had babies often make good birth partners, if you are close to them. They will know most of what you are going through. Again, though, it is important that they are singing from the same hymn sheet as you — in other words, that they know and respect your choices. If your mother feels that her three caesareans were the best thing that ever happened to her, she may not be the best support if you are determined to achieve a vaginal delivery.

For the majority of women nowadays, however, their birth partner is usually their life partner. Today's fathers are, for the most part, very willing participants in their children's births — at least to the extent they can be! They may be the person most in tune with your needs, and they may be able to read signals from you that others cannot. Talk through your needs and expectations with your husband and partner, and ensure that they are happy with the role they will play.

From my own experience, dads are much more relaxed when they know that their partner is getting the special attention of a doula, especially if things get a bit messy. At a recent birth I supported, at one point dad was sitting in the corner with the blood pressure cuff on him, trying to take his own blood pressure! Hospitals with all their high-tech machines are like Toyland to many nervous dads. Once the pressure is off they can really relax and participate in a way that is most comfortable for them. Research shows that dads interact with mums more and touch them more when doulas are present. Doulas help fathers deal with the not-so-pleasant aspects of labour such as blood, pain and sheer unpredictability. Recent evidence has shown that the presence of a doula is associated with fewer medical interventions and shorter births, and that both mothers and babies have a more positive experience.

Post-natal doulas can also be a great help in the early days of parenthood. They can help with breastfeeding, newborn care and help new parents get some well-needed rest. This is especially crucial if the new parents have no family living nearby.

Here's what a good birth partner can do for you:

- Know your needs and be able to pass them on to the midwife or consultant;

- Be informed of everything that might happen during the labour and delivery;

- Be able to help you to relax;

- Reassure you if things seem to be going differently to how you thought they would;

- Help you to make important decisions at the right time, or to stick to your guns if it is in your best interest and that of your baby.

THE FEAR FACTOR

In a world where most first-time mothers' beliefs about birth are formed though horror stories from their mothers, sisters and friends, and endless reruns of reality birth shows, it's no wonder most mothers are terrified of birth and more are choosing to have caesareans. Fear slows labour (see pages 83–85). So how can you get past it?

Get informed: read up on the latest research about natural birth, and read books that accentuate the positive. I highly recommend Ina May Gaskin's *Guide to Childbirth* or Sherri Minelli's *Journey into Motherhood*. Read stories of births that went well — it will change your whole outlook on pregnancy and birth. When someone tries to tell you their horror story, ask them to wait until you've had your baby. Talk to mothers who have had the kind of birth you want. Think about your birth plan, focusing on what you do want rather than what you don't.

YOUR BIRTH PLAN

Planning for your pregnancy and labour isn't easy. For most of us, just planning a night out with the girls takes efforts of military proportions. If you have read ahead and know of the choices you will face during the actual labour, you should have a good idea of what you do and don't want at the hospital. **Birth plans** can be daunting to write, but just keep it short and focus on what is really important to you. Just use bullet points. Some women (and hospitals) don't think birth plans are worth doing, because there are so many unknown factors involved. But that's like saying you can't control the weather, so why bother carrying an umbrella?

A birth plan does not lock you into a position that cannot be changed when circumstances change. It is not a contract between you and your caregiver; nor is it a blueprint for the perfect labour. It is a statement expressing in practical terms what you believe the birth experience should be like for you, in terms of pain relief, positions, interventions, etc., but with the understanding that there are no guarantees.

Indeed, even if you're planning a home birth and know exactly who will be present at the birth, it is worthwhile writing a birth plan. Writing a birth plan helps you to look at every possible situation and consider and discuss what you would like to have happen during your labour and delivery. A birth plan simply opens the lines of communication for you and your caregiver to begin discussing these important issues. The best time to do this is prenatally, *not* at the birth. Don't wait until you are at 38 weeks to start a birth plan discussion — start thinking about it now, whether you're at six weeks or 26 weeks.

During labour, your midwife/consultant or your partner can refer to the birth plan if needs be. For example, if labour is progressing more slowly than expected, and you do not want any artificial augmentation, there should be no need to ask you about it; they simply need to read it in the plan.

I've heard some midwives refer to birth plans as "c-section plans" because there are couples who go to the hospital with very unrealistic birth plans and expectations that are too high and not flexible. It's important that you know what you *do* want out of this experience (assuming your baby is healthy) as well as what you don't. Downloading a birth plan from the web without educating yourself on why you're choosing not to have a particular intervention can turn your birth plan into a ticket to the theatre (and we're not talking about the Gaiety).

Here is a sample birth plan to help you get started. If the only thing you feel strongly about for your birth is to avoid an episiotomy, then just put that in the birth plan and be sure your partner/doula/ consultant/midwife understand and support your wishes. There are also sample birth plans in the chapters on caesarean sections and on home birth.

SAMPLE BIRTH PLAN

We are looking forward to sharing our birth experience with you. We have created this birth plan in order to outline some of our preferences for birth. We would appreciate you reviewing this plan. We understand that there may be situations in which our choices may not be possible, but we hope that you will help us to move toward our goals as much as possible and to make this labour and birth a great experience.

We do not want to replace the medical personnel, but instead want to be informed of any procedures in advance, and to be allowed the chance to give informed consent. Thank you!

I prefer to labour in an upright position (squatting, sitting, etc), on my hands and knees or side lying. I also wish to shower if available, use a **birth ball** and have music during my labour. I realise that the hospital policy may limit these positions with the administration of medications. I wish to drink and eat lightly as desired.

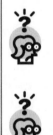

There should be no **artificial rupture of membranes**.

If labour slows down I prefer to change positions or try nipple stimulation before artificial **augmentation**.

I wish to give birth in whatever position I feel most comfortable with.

I prefer not to have an episiotomy unless there is a medical emergency, and would rather tear.

I wish my husband and my doula to remain at my bedside at all times and my husband will accompany me to c-section if that becomes necessary.

I would prefer to allow the cord to stop **pulsating** before cutting it.

Please place the baby on my stomach and allow me to breastfeed as soon as possible. I know that having your newborn on the breast helps shrink the uterus and reduces bleeding.

I would prefer not to be offered pain medication. If I need it I will ask for it.

If I do have an **epidural** I would like the epidural to wear off slightly as I approach full dilation and the pushing stage.

I would prefer not to be coached to push by hospital staff but will push when I have the urge.

If our baby must go to the nursery for evaluation or medical treatment, my husband will accompany our baby at all times.

As I will be breastfeeding, please do not give our baby supplements (including formula, glucose or plain water).

HELPING YOURSELF TO COMPLEMENTARY THERAPIES

Many women in Ireland fully embrace homeopathy, reflexology and seem to be very well versed in other natural "remedies" that may help with pregnancy complaints. This chapter looks at a number of possible aids to pregnancy and birth, including:

- Massage

- Aromatherapy

- Herbs

- Bach Flower Remedies

- Homeopathy

- Active Birth and Yoga

ANTENATAL MASSAGE

Antenatal massage is growing in popularity in Ireland. There is never going to be a better time to enjoy a massage than when you're pregnant. It is sheer bliss and, from personal experience, quite addictive once you try it. Swollen ankles are a thing of the past; back aches just melt away; and your baby also gets the benefits of all those happy hormones (**endorphins**) your brain creates from being really pampered. Antenatal massage therapists use a special table or pad with hollowed out areas to accommodate your belly and, often, your breasts as well, so you can lie face-down. For many of us, being able to lie face-down is a distant memory until after the birth. Some don't have the special tables, so you will lie on your side with several soft pillows to support you. If you haven't had a massage before you can keep your undies on if it makes you more comfortable. A really good massage therapist will be very skilful at keeping you "draped" in all the right places throughout your massage, so you can just focus on relaxing.

BENEFITS OF PREGNANCY MASSAGE

- Emotional support and nurturing touch;

- Relaxation and decreased insomnia;

- Stress relief on weight-bearing joints, such as ankles, lower back and pelvis;

- Neck and back pain relief caused by muscle imbalance and weakness;

- Assistance in maintaining proper posture;

- Preparing the muscles used during childbirth;

- Reduced swelling in hands and feet;

- Lessened sciatic pain;

- Fewer leg cramps;

- Headache and sinus congestion relief.
  © www.pregnancytoday.com. Reproduced with kind permission.

AROMATHERAPY IN PREGNANCY

Although there has been no scientific research into the benefits of aromatherapy during pregnancy, women who are familiar with this holistic therapy before pregnancy often find it beneficial during pregnancy too. The smell of an apple tart baking can transport you back to Saturday afternoons at your Nan's house and instantly give you a feeling of comfort and wellbeing. Aromatherapy is all about using smells (aromas) to bring about physiological and emotional changes. We don't really understand how aromatherapy works, but our sense of smell is one of our most powerful senses. You've probably noticed that your sense of smell has really heightened during pregnancy and it will be even more evident during labour. Not all essential oils are safe to use during pregnancy; read all instructions carefully, and talk to a professional aromatherapist.

Morning Sickness

To help prevent morning sickness, www.thebabyorchard.com recommends that you "diffuse petitgrain and mandarin oils in an electric vaporiser overnight or sprinkle the oils on a tissue to place by your bedside as you sleep". For me the only thing that could keep away the nausea was the smell of lemons. I would carry a bag of chopped-up lemons with me everywhere. I'm sure I looked very strange standing in the supermarket with my face in a plastic ziplock bag sniffing lemons . . . but, hey, whatever worked.

Tired and Emotional

If you are exhausted or very emotional, www.thebabyorchard.com recommends that you "choose balancing lavender, geranium or bergamot oil for your diffuser". Even if you don't have essential oils at home there's a huge selection of products now that come with added lavender. A nice warm lavender bath can make your day.

Massage

The benefits of massage have already been outlined; add in a safe, relaxing essential oil to the mix, and you're in heaven! During the first three months, www.thebabyorchard.com recommends using "plain sweet almond oil or another carrier", especially if you suffer from morning, noon and night sickness. Lavender is a universal scent for calming the senses and can be used for a nice soak in the bathtub in the evening, especially if you are suffering from insomnia. Aromatherapy is growing in popularity as a tool for birth to help mum stay relaxed (anything has to be better than the smell of antiseptic). If you are planning on using essential oils during your birth, let your caregiver know.

Safety

Again, it must be stressed that not all oils are safe to use during pregnancy; check all labels and talk to your aromatherapist. Here's www.thebabyorchard.com again: "For use on the skin or in the bath, dilute essential oils using a maximum of two drops of essential oil per 10 ml (two teaspoonfuls) of carrier oil. Do not use neat essential oils on the skin."

HERBAL USE FOR PREGNANCY AND BIRTH

The use of herbs during pregnancy and birth goes back hundreds of years when the "wise women" of the villages would create preparations for mothers based on recipes passed down through time. These were the earliest forms of medicine. Herbs are perceived as "natural" but their potency should not be underestimated, especially during pregnancy. It's very important not to self-prescribe any kind of medicine for yourself while pregnant, whether it's natural or over-the-counter, unless it comes from a reliable source. (I would not consider the internet a reliable source.)

There has been very limited research into the side effects of traditional herbal remedies although this probably has more to do with the fact that drug companies would not be interested in sponsoring such research; but there are many experienced midwives who swear by them. Herbs affect different women in different ways, so it's very important to seek the expertise of a qualified herbalist who specialises in remedies for pregnant and/or breastfeeding mums.

At some point in your pregnancy, someone may well ask you if you have started your raspberry leaf tea yet. This is a herbal tea that is thought to tone the muscles of the uterus, but the research has been limited to a few small studies in Australia. Over the last year or two, RLT has become a staple for many women in Ireland, often taken with the mistaken belief that downing bucketfuls of this woeful-tasting "tea" will get labour underway. You're more likely to end up with some serious bathroom visits rather than the desired outcome.

Please let your midwife and/or doctor know if you are taking any kind of herbs during your pregnancy and labour.

For more information about herbs and pregnancy, including herbs to use during birth, to improve lactation, and to help the newborn infant, see *Wise Woman Herbal for the Childbearing Year* by Susan Weed (Ash Tree Publishing).

BACH FLOWER REMEDIES

Another wonderful tool that is safe to use at any time during pregnancy and birth are the Bach flower remedies (or essences). The flower remedies were discovered by Dr Edward Bach in the 1920s and are a safe, natural way of dealing with the negative emotions that he believed were the cause of illness. The remedies harmonise your mental state and enable you to think more positively. Some of the most used remedies are:

- *Mimulus*: A useful remedy if you feel afraid of the birth or pain or fear of there being something wrong with the baby.

- *Elm*: This is a great remedy if you feel doubtful of your ability to cope and are feeling overwhelmed and stressed.

- *Mustard*: For unexplained depression. Great for the baby blues.

- *Olive* is a must for the fatigue that so often comes during the first and third trimester.

- *Rescue Remedy*: This is the ideal remedy for labour to help ease panic and shock! It is a very calming remedy. A drop of Rescue Remedy rubbed onto your baby can also help him adjust to the shock of life outside the womb. Rescue Remedy cream can also be used on sore nipples. Apply as often as necessary. Before a feed, simply wipe the excess residue from your nipples.

Bach flower remedies are preserved in brandy, but the recommended dosage is two drops in a glass of water, so don't expect to get a buzz from the Bach flowers. You'd probably ingest the same amount of alcohol walking by the Guinness Brewery! If you're concerned about taking any alcohol during your pregnancy then just keep this in mind. There hasn't been any research conducted on the safety or effectiveness of Bach Flower Remedies during pregnancy and birth.

HOMEOPATHY

Homeopathy is very popular in Ireland. All over the country women are comparing prices of arnica at their antenatal appointments and debating the best places to get their "labour kit". According to the World Health Organisation, homeopathy is the second most widely used form of medicine in the world.

How Does It Work?

Your homeopath will recommend certain "remedies" for you to take (often in the form of tiny sugar pills) depending on the symptoms you have. The treatments are based on the idea that a remedy can help a problem if it produces symptoms similar to the ailment (this is known as the "Law of Similars"). As homeopathy is quite safe, you can use it for children, adults and animals. The remedies themselves are made from minute plant and mineral extracts. Keep any strong-smelling aromatherapy oils away from your homeopathic remedies or they will lose their potency. Of course, it is wise to let your caregiver know if you are taking any homeopathic remedies and also to let your homeopath know if you're on any medication.

Some Uses for Homeopathy during Birth:

- Induction: Caulophyllum and Cimicifuga (please consult with your caregiver before attempting any kind of induction);

- Turning a breech baby: Pulsatilla is a favourite (for more on breech birth, see pages 121–123);

- Arnica should be in every mother's birth bag; it's great for preventing bruising and can help you heal faster.

There are thousands of homeopathic remedies available. Have a consultation with a qualified homeopath so you can get the remedy that will have the most beneficial effect for you. You should *never* self-prescribe.

ACTIVE BIRTH OR YOGA CLASSES

The object of *active birth* classes is to help you use movement and gravity to labour in a natural and effective way. *Active birth* is when a mother instinctively moves into positions that help her cope with labour, by using natural position changes and gravity to help the baby through the birth canal. It should not be confused with "active management", which is the term used for a third party (your doctor or midwife) who manages your labour. Gentle movement in labour can ease pain and also help labour progress. Active birth classes borrow heavily from yoga techniques, adapted for pregnancy.

ACTIVE BIRTH CLASSES: WHAT'S INVOLVED

Classes typically begin with stretches to increase flexibility, and you may then practise movements for use in labour. For example, you might stand upright and sway your hips, or kneel on all fours and move your hips in larger or smaller circles to relieve imaginary contractions. You will pay attention to your breathing during all movements and stretches — nothing complicated; you simply focus on breathing out in a slow and controlled fashion.

It is important to practise these movements and breathing techniques often and regularly. The best way to do this is to attend classes as often as possible; this is much more effective than simply attending one class or workshop on breathing techniques and hoping you can remember them when you are in labour.

When you have practised these movements so often that they become second nature, you may well find yourself automatically using them in labour. Because the movements and breathing patterns are simple, and you have practised them often, they can be very effective tools to help you labour.

Active birth teachers and antenatal yoga teachers practise in most areas of Ireland; classes are normally held weekly.

© www.homebirth.org. Adapted and reproduced with kind permission.

GENTLE EXERCISES DURING PREGNANCY

Although you don't want to start a new exercise regime while pregnant, pregnancy isn't an excuse to lie on the couch for nine months. Staying active and fit during pregnancy will help you feel better and can even help shorten your labour. When exercising during pregnancy, you should:

- Avoid exercises that require you to lie on your back, such as sit-ups, after your twentieth week.

- Avoid exercising in very hot weather.

- Drink lots of water.

- Wear a good sports bra that supports your breasts.

- Never exercise to the point of exhaustion.

- Do **Kegel exercises** (or pelvic floor exercises) religiously. The pelvic floor supports the bladder, uterus, and intestines. The added weight of the uterus during pregnancy can stretch out that floor, causing either the intestines or bladder to drop down. This is one of the reasons that so many elderly women suffer from incontinence. Prevention is the best medicine. Kegels involve contracting and releasing the PF muscles, similarly to stopping the flow of urination. Tighten and relax the muscle quickly several times a day.

- Call a doctor if you develop serious symptoms, such as pain, dizziness, vaginal bleeding or fluid leaking from the vagina.

Pelvic Rock

This exercise is good for lower back ache. To do the exercise, get on your hands and knees and slowly arch your back like an angry cat, tilting your pelvis. Hold it for a moment; then relax your back to a normal position. Sometimes just wiggling your hips in this position can feel wonderful.

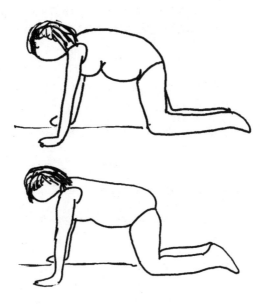

Tailor Pose

Sit comfortably on the floor and bring the soles of your feet together pressing down lightly on your thighs so you feel a gentle stretch.

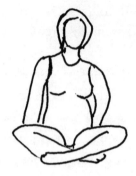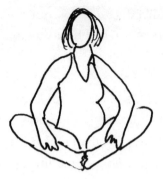

All Illustrations © Janelle Durham (www.janelledurham.com)

LABOUR: IS THIS IT?

You've imagined this day for a long time and now you're wondering, *"Is this it?"* If you are a first-time mum, then you may have a few false alarms and be worried that you won't know if you are really in labour. This chapter describes some of the usual signs that things are starting to happen and labour is about to get under way. Sometimes things will happen at once, while for other mothers labour gets underway more gradually. But no matter how your labour begins, staying as relaxed as possible will help things progress much more quickly and less stressfully.

Don't be surprised if in the last few days of your pregnancy your energy comes back in bursts. You may have what some mothers refer to as the "nesting instinct". You may feel the need to get things organised and clean the house from top to bottom; this is very normal, so let your partner know you haven't totally lost the plot!

LABOUR: RECOGNISING THE SIGNS

In the first stage of labour, the cervix dilates from a closed position to 10 cm, when it is said to be fully dilated. In most Irish hospitals you are not "officially" in labour until you reach 3 cm. If you get to the hospital and are less than 3 cm, if everything else is as it should be, the best thing to do is to go home and relax; check this with your hospital. It can take up to 12 hours for the cervix to become fully dilated, although this is very individual; some mothers dilate more quickly than others.

Contractions

What are they?

Contractions are regular tightenings of the uterine muscles and occur throughout labour. During the first stage, these contractions help to dilate the cervix. In the second stage, they help to push the baby down the birth canal and in the third stage, the contractions also help deliver the placenta. When your contractions start, many first-time mothers mistakenly believe that they need to do 50 laps around the block to keep things moving and then find they are exhausted two hours into labour!

For labour to progress, it is important to reduce the adrenaline in your system; physical activity and stress increase adrenaline and reduce the "feel-good" hormones (endorphins). For more on this, see pages 82–85. In the early stages especially, try to conserve your energy and relax as much as possible. If you're a first-time mother, this is going to be hard because of all the excitement; that's why it's so important to practise some relaxation techniques long before you go into labour. For any birth partners reading this, it's up to you to help mum stay relaxed. Turn down the lights, run a warm bath for your partner or get the shower going — and above all, stay calm.

How do they feel?

Women experience contractions in a variety of different ways. Some say that they feel like very bad period pains in the stomach. Others describe the feeling as that of extreme constipation and wind. Sometimes, contractions appear to originate from the back and radiate towards the front. Contractions may also be accompanied by backache, nausea and/or diarrhoea. If you're having a homebirth, call your midwife and let her know what's going on.

What do I do?

If the contractions get regular and more frequent, increasing in intensity, call the hospital or contact your midwife as you may be in labour. Have a bath or shower, dim the lights and relax.

How do I time contractions?

When timing contractions, you need to be aware of two things: how frequent and how strong the contractions are. Start the timer when you get the first contraction. The time when it ends is used to determine the duration of the contraction. When the second contraction starts, use the interval between the start time of this contraction and the start time of the previous contraction to determine the frequency of contractions.

Remember that many people wrongly time contractions as the interval between the end time of the first and the start time of the next contraction.

In a first pregnancy, the cervix is closed throughout pregnancy. As labour begins (usually unnoticed) your cervix begins to efface (thin out) and dilate (open) when it is ripe and ready for your baby to be born.

A "Birth Show"

What is it?

A protective plug of mucous seals the cervix at the neck of the uterus throughout pregnancy. This plug begins to come away and passes down the vagina as a bloodstained, mucous discharge. This is called a "show".

When does it happen?

A show may occur several days before labour or it may even occur during the first stage of labour.

Your Membranes Release

Throughout pregnancy your baby floats in a sac containing amniotic fluid, or "bag of waters". When your baby is ready to be born, the membranes of this amniotic sac release causing the amniotic fluid to flow out of the vagina.

What will I feel?

You will either feel the fluid trickling or a sudden gush of fluid out through the vagina. Most commonly, there is a trickle if the baby has engaged by this time and its head has the same effect as a cork in a bottle.

When does it happen?

Your waters may release or "break" several hours before the onset of labour or this may occur during labour itself. For some women their waters will release and labour doesn't kick in for a while; this is normal. You don't have to worry about your baby; your body continues to produce amniotic fluid. Some babies are even born "in the caul" (the waters don't release until the moment the baby is being born). If your membranes release before 37 weeks, however, you should contact your caregiver immediately.

What to do?

If the fluid is clear, wear a sanitary towel if it makes you feel more comfortable. Call your midwife or the hospital. If the fluid is greenish, yellow or brown in colour, it may be a sign that the baby is in distress. This coloured fluid is actually due to the baby having passed meconium, its first stool, which would normally not happen until after birth. Call your midwife or hospital immediately.

Going to the Hospital

Staying home as long as you are comfortable is a great idea. Being in your own environment will help you deal with labour much better than being in the strange environment of the hospital with bright lights, noise and strangers. You'll feel much more relaxed at home, which is essential for helping your labour progress. If at any time you feel that something isn't quite right or have bleeding or your waters change colour, go to the hospital, or call your midwife if you're having a home-birth. Most hospitals recommend coming in once contractions are consistent and lasting at least 60 seconds every five to seven minutes. Your partner should bear in mind the distance from the hospital and traffic conditions, especially if you think you may need to leave for the hospital in the early morning or evening rush hour. It might not be a bad idea to do a "dry run" to the hospital some evening and see how long it takes you (partners: keep the car filled up!).

Premature Labour

What is it?

When labour starts before 37 weeks of pregnancy, it is termed as premature labour.

Why does it happen?

A history of premature birth, high temperature, or a multiple pregnancy all contribute to a premature labour. Unfortunately, premature labour is hard to predict.

How will I recognise the signs?

The signs of a premature labour are more or less similar to real full-term labour, as discussed above. It also depends on the prematurity of the labour; if you are close to 37 weeks, signs will be almost identical to a proper labour, whereas if you are many weeks behind, you may experience just a low back pain with or without contractions.

How is the baby affected in a premature labour?

Most babies born before 24 weeks won't survive. However, if born between 24 and 30 weeks, your baby will be very immature but will be able to survive in a special care unit. If your baby is born anytime after 34 weeks, he may be able to survive even without special care. If your caregiver is successful in stopping premature labour, you may be advised to either stay in hospital or at home on strict bedrest.

A premature baby's lungs are very immature and can cause major problems as the lungs don't know how to breathe. If there is a risk of your baby being born prematurely, steroids may be given to you which reach across to the baby through the placenta and help the baby's lungs to develop rapidly.

What happens if I go into premature labour?

- Attempts may be made to stop the contractions temporarily, either through the use of drugs for 48 hours or through antibiotics if you have an infection with a high temperature.

- You may be given an injection (such as pethidine) to calm you down.

- If you are dehydrated, a drip may be given to replenish your fluids.

- You will be advised to take steroids to speed up the development of your baby's lungs; this takes 24 hours to take effect.

- A premature labour is much quicker than a full-term labour, mainly because the baby is smaller.

© *Adapted and reproduced with the kind permission of www.mothersbliss.com*

WHAT TO BRING TO THE HOSPITAL

A lot of mums live in the hope they'll go early. So the bags are packed and ready to go by the sixth month, if not sooner! Only five per cent of babies are born on their "guess date". It's probably a good idea to have your bags ready by 37 weeks, which is considered to be full term (anywhere between 37 and 42 weeks).

For Mum

- This book

- Birth plan (have a few copies)

- Light dressing gown

- Lip balm

- Hair scrunchies or clips

- Antibacterial wipes (especially if you're sharing a bathroom with four other new mums)

- Flipflops (same reason as the wipes)

- Breast pads

- Slippers

- Two pairs of socks (you might not need them because hospitals are usually very warm)

- Old nightie (not essential as you'll be given a gown anyway, but it's nice to be in your own clothes)

- Three pairs of pyjamas, or a couple of tracksuits (you'll feel better being dressed)

- Toothbrush and toothpaste

- Shampoo and conditioner

- Deodorant

- Shower gel

- Two packs of sanitary towels (industrial strength with wings) or maternity pads

- Two towels

- Sponge or face cloth

- Big old granny knickers or disposables

- CD player, CDs and earphones

- Eye mask

- Going home outfit (something loose and comfy)

- Snacks — energy bars for labour and drinks

- Rescue remedy

- Arnica

- Lansinoh cream for breastfeeding

- A good nursing bra and a pair of pyjamas designed for breast-feeding

- Change for the phone.

Baby

- Car seat

- Six vests

- Six babygrows

- Five bibs

- Two soft towels

- One pack of newborn nappies

- Soother (not recommended if you are breastfeeding to avoid nipple confusion)

- Cotton wool

- Sudocreme

- Scratch mits and hat

- Outfit and blanket for going home (partner can bring this in on the day you leave).

Partner

- Fill up the car with petrol

- Change for parking

- Mobile phone (with credit)

- List of numbers

- Camera and film

- Sandwiches and snacks (fruit bars).

INDUCTION

There can be many varied reasons for your care provider wanting to induce your labour. In Ireland the rates vary from 10 per cent to a whopping 45 per cent! If your doctor spots any signs of pre-eclampsia (high blood pressure and protein in your urine), he or she may well recommend induction, as the risks of waiting may be too high. Other reasons for induction can include if your pregnancy goes over 40 weeks (most hospitals will be fine waiting 10–14 days past your guess date — see below) or if your waters break and you haven't gone into labour within a certain timeframe. There can be other reasons for a medical induction, such as health complications of the mother, but those are the most common.

When You Are Overdue

So 40 weeks have come and gone; you feel like you've been pregnant forever; no shows, no leaks and not a single contraction. Eviction is starting to look appealing.

Your estimated due date (EDD) is just that — an estimate — it is not an appointment! It is based on a nineteenth-century formula called Naegele's Rule, which assumes that ovulation occurs on day 14 of a 28-day cycle for all women. We now know this to be incorrect. Your baby is considered to be full term anywhere from 37–42 weeks. Only 5 per cent of babies are born on their due date. Women generally assume they are overdue once they go past 40 weeks, but they are not actually overdue until reaching 42 weeks.

When you are already past your estimated due date (EDD), your care provider may suggest inducing your labour. Remember that only five per cent of babies are born on their due date. Some care providers suggest inductions based on the size of your baby. Ultrasounds are notoriously inaccurate. Think how difficult it is to estimate the weight of a baby you are physically holding — now try it with a black and white photo! Contrary to popular belief, the camera doesn't add 10 lbs — especially to ultrasound images!

Although it's very tempting to know exactly when your baby will be born, inductions should never be done if the reason is that you are tired of being pregnant or want to have your baby on a specific date or simply for the convenience of a doctor's holiday schedule. An induction comes with varied risks, depending on what type of stimulant is used to attempt to induce labour. Usually you can find out if you are a good candidate for induction by having your doctor give you a **Bishop Score**. This is a system that takes into account the position of the baby, the softness and readiness of your cervix, as well as the position of your cervix, to rate if an induction is more or less likely to work. It is recommended that an induction only take place if your Bishop Score is above 9.

Inductions are generally more painful than "normal" labour as your body doesn't have the ability to adjust to the natural start of labour. Your endorphins don't have a chance to catch up to labour that has been artificially started.

Induction Methods

In consultation with your care provider, you can use "natural induction methods" or medical induction methods. It is not recommended to try natural induction methods before reaching 40 weeks, and you should always discuss any method you want to try with your care provider before attempting it. In fact, "natural" is a bit of a misnomer. Any form of induction, whether it is "natural" or not, is an attempt to artificially kickstart labour. You will probably get lots of "advice" from your friends on the best way to do this, including sex, acupuncture, eating spicy food, walking, eating fresh pineapple . . . the list goes on. And it may seem like some of these methods work, but there's no proof that Auntie Orla wouldn't have gone into labour anyway, even if she hadn't cleaned out the local takeaway of their Madras "special"!

Here are how some common induction medications work, as well as their risks and possible side effects:

- **Prostaglandins**: Artificial hormones used to soften the cervix so that it is ready for labour. Risks include possible hyperstimulation of the uterus and possible **foetal distress**, which could lead to a c-section.

- **Oxytocin** (also known as *syntocinon* or *pitocin* or *pit*): This drug is given by IV in order to make the uterus start contracting. It is routinely used to speed up labour in some hospitals. Side effects of pitocin can include: hyperstimulation of the uterus, foetal distress, oxygen deprivation resulting in low **Apgar scores** at birth, blood loss and jaundice. In first-time mothers, the use of pitocin increases the likelihood of having a c-section.

- **Stripping or sweeping your membranes**: Beginning at your 38-week appointment, your care provider may suggest a vaginal exam every week to gauge the progress of your cervix and to check to see if you are dilated at all. While this can give you hope (if you are slightly dilated) that you will go into labour soon, it is no real indication of when labour will start. Sometimes you will be 1–2 cm dilated for weeks before going into labour. Sometimes during these vaginal exams, your doctor may strip or **sweep your membranes** (with your consent of course). What this means is that he/she may (if you are more than a small fingertip dilated) sweep their finger around the inside of your cervix to separate your bag of waters from the entrance to your cervix. This is believed to release your body's natural prostaglandins in order to possibly start labour. While this may sound like a great idea if you are feeling ready to not be pregnant anymore, make sure to ask your doctor if they routinely do this procedure and ask them not to do it to you. Your risk of infection increases with any foreign object being inserted into your vagina. It is also possible to rupture your membranes accidentally, which comes with its own complications.

It is very important when selecting a caregiver that you are comfortable with his/her induction policies. If you are considering an induction it is important to understand the risks involved. Starting the induction process on a mother whose body is not ready to give birth can cause more problems than it solves. Midwives and doulas often describe a "cascade of intervention" when the natural flow of the birthing process is disrupted (see page 114). One intervention leads to another and often the end result is what you were originally trying to avoid — a caesarean.

PAIN MANAGEMENT IN LABOUR

Although the epidural is often described in degrees of bliss, there is no perfect drug. All drugs have the potential to affect you and your baby. It's ironic that we spend nine months swearing off drink, cigarettes, coffee and even hairdye and then we want the epidural waiting in the car park! When considering your options, think about how you currently deal with pain. When you have a headache, do you immediately reach for the paracetamol, or do you take a nice bath or have your partner rub your head?

In general, women think of labour pain as one continuous excruciating ordeal. This is reinforced by comments from friends such as "You don't get a medal for not taking the drugs". However, labour pain is not like the pain you get when you break your leg. Breaking down the contractions makes it much more manageable. Let's say you're well into active labour and things are progressing perfectly. Even at the height of your contractions, chances are you'll be having a 90-second contraction every five minutes. That sounds like a lot, but let's break it down. The contraction is made up of three stages: the build-up, the peak and the release. In a 90-second contraction, the first 30 seconds are when you feel the contraction starting to build. Take a nice deep breath and you can focus all of your attention on the next 30 seconds — the "peak". After those 30 seconds are over, the contraction ebbs away and you can rest for another five minutes. So essentially you only have to deal with severe pain for 30 seconds, every five minutes. In one hour, that is 12 contractions multiplied by 30 second "peaks", which is only six minutes each hour that you really have to focus on. And the contractions usually only get that intense towards the end! Is that so awful?

METHODS OF MANAGING PAIN

Epidural

Getting an **epidural** can in itself be an exercise in futility, depending on which hospital you're in. You'll be warned by everyone: don't get it too early . . . and don't get it too late! To "get" the epidural, you will have to sit or lie with your back curved (like the hunchback) while an anaesthetist inserts a **catheter** into your back (see page 104). You have to remain completely still for this procedure, which can take up to twenty minutes — not exactly easy when you're having a contraction. As soon as you feel one coming on, tell the anaesthetist and he will stop until it's over. Your partner might do well to sit in front of you and hold your hand; watching an epidural procedure can make you queasy.

The epidural is not just a quick needle in the back. Once you've had the first intervention of an epidural there are others that follow suit: you have to have a drip to keep your blood pressure up; you have to be continuously monitored, and you will most likely be on your back for a considerable length of time. Ask the midwives to shift you on to your side every hour or so. It is ironic that throughout pregnancy mothers are advised *not* to sleep on their backs because it can restrict the blood flow to the baby — and yet that's how you end up sometimes for a long time when you have an epidural! Another common side effect from epidurals that is still "in the closet" so to speak is that once every muscle in your body has been anaesthetised you cannot control any excess gas that needs to exit — so prepare for some rippers! Don't worry, though, it's quite normal, even if it is quite mortifying when you aren't expecting it.

The epidural has been equally praised and damned by labouring women. For some, it is a positive experience, the pain relief allowing for a more relaxed birth experience. For others, however, the loss of control can be frustrating at best, and for some the epidural slows down and complicates what might otherwise be a straightforward labour. Some mothers lose the urge to push and have to have a vacuum or forceps delivery. Some mothers can develop a fever.

Babies are also affected by epidurals. Often the decision to accept an epidural is made without an awareness of these and other significant risks to both mother and baby. These risks are explained in more detail in the next chapter (pages 105–106).

Narcotic Analgesics

While the epidural is a locally acting anaesthetic, narcotic painkillers such as pethidine act to reduce the entire body's sense of pain.

Pethidine is the most common drug given in Irish hospitals. It works very much like morphine. It is usually given as an injection in the thigh or buttock, or sometimes as a drip, takes about twenty minutes to start working and lasts about two to three hours. Pethidine can make you sleepy and trippy. The problem with pethidine, apart from its side effects (see below) is that it seems to affect women in different ways. For some, the pain relief is minimal, or may only work early in labour, while others can be left feeling totally spaced out, distressed or feeling a complete lack of control.

Specific risks of pethidine include:

- It can cause nausea;

- You may need a drip;

- It can slow labour causing a need for pitocin/syntocinon to speed it up again (which increases your risk of caesarean);

- You'll need continuous foetal monitoring, which decreases your mobility (probably not a bad thing if you're tripping on pethidine anyway);

- Like any drug, it might not work;

- It affects the baby both before he's born and after through your breastmilk, so he may not show any interest in breastfeeding.

If your labour is progressing normally you probably won't have the option of pethidine if you are getting close to actually giving birth because the drug can affect the baby's breathing. Your body's natural endorphins are 200 times stronger than morphine, and come with no negative side effects — see below.

Taking the Edge Off: Entonox (Gas and Air)

Entonox, commonly known as "gas and air", is a mild painkiller consisting of oxygen and nitrous oxide, inhaled through a mask or mouthpiece. When you feel a contraction coming on, you take a nice deep breath and by the time the contraction peaks you should have some relief; it doesn't completely take the pain away but will take the edge off. If you find it makes you queasy or dizzy you can just stop using it. There has been little research done on the long-term effects of gas and air on mothers and babies.

TENS Machine (Transcutaneous Electrical Nerve Stimulation)

Transcutaneous means "through the skin". **TENS** machines (available for rent in Boots Chemists) deliver small electrical pulses to the body via electrodes placed on the skin. The sticky patches are placed on your back. It looks like those tummy-trimming devices that were popular a few years ago. Think of it like internet broadband — your spinal cord can only carry so much information to the brain and if its capacity is used up with electrical stimulation from the TENS machine, there's no room for the pain signals to get through. TENS doesn't work for everyone; some mothers find it very distracting, but at least it's self-administered and you can turn it up as you need it. If you don't like it, you can just take off the patches. There are no known side effects to using TENS, but you have to wonder if applying electrodes to your body affects the brain and that precise orchestration of hormone release that helps birth progress.

THE SECRET TO AN EASIER BIRTH: HOW YOUR HORMONES AFFECT BIRTH

To make birth easier and labour shorter, it's critical to ensure the birth hormones are encouraged to do their job effectively. Four major hormonal systems are active during labour and birth. These involve oxytocin, the "hormone of love" (Michel Odent); endorphins, the "feel good" hormones; adrenaline, hormones of excitement and stress; and prolactin, the mothering hormone. These hormones are common to all mammals. For birth to proceed easily the primitive (instinctive) brain must take over from the front part of your brain (the thinking part). This occurs naturally and is helped by an atmosphere of quiet and privacy, with dim lighting and little conversation or distractions. Under these conditions, a mother will instinctively choose the movements, sounds, breathing, and positions that will birth her baby most easily. Creating this atmosphere in hospital isn't easy, but a CD player with calming music and an eye mask can be very helpful.

Endorphins and high levels of adrenaline cannot co-exist in labour. If there is an excess of adrenaline, then the body's own painkillers (endorphins) are not present. Likewise if endorphin levels are increased, adrenaline levels lower, which makes for a much more comfortable labour.

Oxytocin

Oxytocin is the hormone that sends signals to your body to start contracting. It has also been shown to affect how we bond with others. Right as your baby is about to be born you have the highest levels of oxytocin in your body than at any other time in your life.

Endorphins

Your body's natural pain relievers are more powerful than morphine (and pethidine). Like oxytocin, endorphins are secreted from the pituitary gland, and high levels are present during sex, pregnancy, birth and breastfeeding. Beta-endorphin is also a stress hormone, released under conditions of duress and pain, when it acts as an analgesic.

Fight-or-Flight Hormones

The hormones adrenaline and noradrenaline are also known as the fight-or-flight hormones or, collectively, as catecholamines. They are secreted in response to stresses such as fright and anxiety, as well as excitement, when they activate the sympathetic nervous system for "fight or flight". We've all experienced this "fight or flight" phenomenon. Millions of years ago, it helped us survive attacks by wild animals. Obviously, for most of us that's no longer a threat, but it's a part of our primitive brain that remains with us. Your body has a physical response to a fright, whether it's real or imagined. How many of us have driven over the speed limit and then spotted a garda car behind us, lights flashing? Remember how your breathing increased . . . your heart raced . . . your hands became sweaty . . . and you probably felt physically sick for a few seconds . . . then the garda car overtook you, speeding off after someone else! While you were reading this your breathing rate probably went up too; the very thought of this scenario created a physical response. That's the effect of adrenaline on the body.

In the first stage of labour, high stress levels inhibit oxytocin production, thereby slowing labour. Adrenaline also acts to reduce blood flow to the uterus and placenta, and therefore to the baby, because the uterus is not a defensive organ. Reduced blood flow means muscles tire quickly. For animals giving birth in the wild, this response is important — the presence of danger would activate this sympathetic response and stop labour until the animal has moved to a safe place to birth or the threat has passed. Unfortunately, the subconscious mind does not differentiate between real and perceived fears for humans, so for most mothers the fight-or-flight response is redundant in labour. You're in a vulnerable position; you can't fight and you can't flee. So your body does the next best thing — it freezes. You may have heard the term "FTP", or failure to progress . . . In humans, high levels of adrenaline are associated with longer labour and adverse foetal heart rate patterns.

After an undisturbed labour, right as the baby is about to be born, these hormones act in a different way. There is a sudden increase in adrenaline levels, which activates the foetal ejection reflex, allowing the baby to be born in a few strong, uncontrollable contractions.

Ways to Optimise the Benefits of your Birth Hormones

Because the slightest disturbance can affect the delicate balance of hormones during birth, the following are essential to help labour progress easily and quickly:

- Anything that helps you stay relaxed during your pregnancy is helpful (e.g. meditation, visualisation or yoga), particularly if you have been practising them over weeks or months.

- Create an atmosphere where you feel safe, unobserved and free to follow your own instincts.

- Reduce physical activity. Activity increases adrenaline in the body which leaves no room for those feel-good hormones. Don't fall into the trap of walking a marathon in labour unless you feel like walking. Being upright has the benefit of helping your baby into a good position, but follow your body's lead — nobody else's. If it feels good to walk, then walk.

- Reduce mental stimulation by keeping lighting low and keeping questions and distractions to a minimum (bring your CD player and eye mask). Relaxation is key.

© Sarah Buckley, www.sarahjbuckley.com. Adapted and reproduced with kind permission from an article by Sarah Buckley MD

PHYSICAL COMFORT MEASURES

What is the first thing you do if you feel a headache coming on? Do you go straight for the painkillers, or do you change what you were doing, sit back and relax first? Similarly, during labour, often a simple change of position, or the use of specific techniques can offer effective pain relief. You may need some prompting to remind you of your techniques (usually the birth partner's starring role).

Position Changes

It is not natural to lie down and stay still when you are uncomfortable. Think of the last time you stubbed your toe; instinctively you probably hopped around swearing like a trooper and rubbing it furiously. The same principles apply in birth. You will instinctively get into positions that feel best for you. Certain positions help the baby to move through the birth canal; move around until you feel an easing of pain. There are other positions which are specifically aimed at reducing pain during back labour (i.e. when the baby is in the posterior position). Remember, if you are having a drug-free birth your body will tell you what to do; you just have to follow its lead. Of course, certain interventions may mean your position is restricted; if you have an epidural, for instance, you will be confined to bed (on your back or on your side).

 Ways to be Active During Labour

The following illustrations are examples of what a mother will instinctively do during labour. Only move about if you feel you need to, not because someone suggests it. Sometimes when the baby is moving down through the pelvis he may put pressure on a certain muscle or nerve. You will automatically counter that pressure by changing position. So there's no need to memorise positions; you'll just do it!

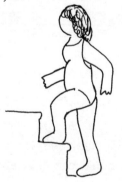 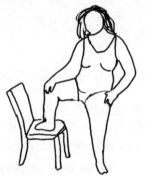

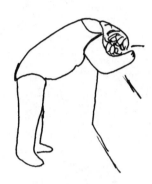
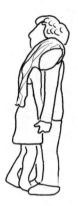
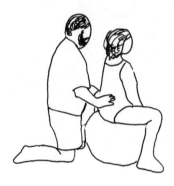

Birth balls are great to have before birth, just to sit on and rock; during birth to help the pelvis open up and take the pressure off the perineum; and after birth to bounce on with your baby and tone up your stomach muscles. During labour you can sit on the ball and have your partner massage your lower back.

All Illustrations © Janelle Durham (www.janelledurham.com)

Positions for Resting During Labour

Just like nobody has ever taught you how to sleep comfortably — in labour you'll automatically get yourself into the best position to rest. Follow your body's lead.

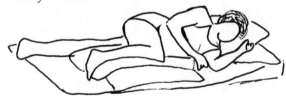

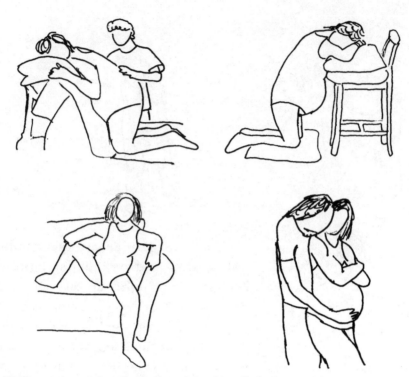

All Illustrations © Janelle Durham (www.janelledurham.com)

Positions for Back Labour (Posterior Baby)

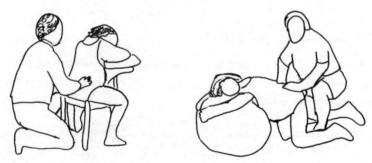

Drape your shoulders and chest over the ball and you can move your hips easily. This is a great position for a woman who is having back labour as the birth partner can apply firm counterpressure to mum's back (she'll tell you how much).

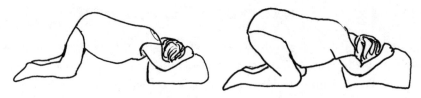

All Illustrations © Janelle Durham (www.janelledurham.com)

Water Birth

Unfortunately, **water birth** is not an option in most Irish hospitals, but is for home births (see pages 157–160). Our Lady of Lourdes in Drogheda and Cavan Hospital do have this option available. The Rotunda is also in the process of getting a pool installed for mothers to labour in, which is good news for mothers in the Dublin area. For some women, there is nothing like the support and comfort of warm water to help them relax and cope with contractions during labour. It is often referred to as the midwife's epidural!

Even if you are not opting for a water birth, make as much use of baths and showers as you can. So if you find water to be relaxing, the best advice is to stay home as long as you can and enjoy the comforts of your own home.

Massage

During some stages of labour, massage can bring welcome relief to the intensity of the contractions. Some women can't bear to have anyone touch them, especially in the late stages of labour. Partners should take the same approach that (hopefully) they have been using throughout the pregnancy, using long, firm strokes following the guidance of your partner.

Using Pain Management Techniques

Even with all the planning in the world, your labour and birth may well pull a few surprises for you, and you need to expect the unexpected. For example, if you want an epidural, you may have to wait a while until you get it, depending on the hospital and where you are in the queue. If your baby decides to come on a Sunday you may not have the option of an epidural.

The best piece of advice you can take is to *listen to what your body is trying to tell you.* If you feel better standing up, then stand up. If you find massage to be too distracting, ask your birth partner to stop. Pain is the body's way of saying *stop!* If you sat on the couch and your leg went numb you would automatically move it. In labour you'll do the same; you won't have to think consciously about a list of practised positions, you'll just do what feels good at particular points in labour — and what feels good for a while may not work as the labour progresses. Some mothers feel lots of rectal pressure (in your bum) as the baby moves down. It's usually only momentarily, and it's a very good sign.

HypnoBirthing®

HypnoBirthing® is a unique antenatal programme that teaches simple but specific self-hypnosis and relaxation techniques for an easier, more gentle birth. HypnoBirthing is not about "training" you to give birth; you innately know how to do that. It's about training your mind to relax so your body can easily do what it was designed for. We haven't lost the ability to birth instinctively, but we have lost the ability to relax so completely that birth can happen more easily, more quickly and often with significantly reduced pain. How many of us really do any relaxation (both mental and physical) on a daily basis? With HypnoBirthing, you'll discover that severe pain does *not* have to be a part of a normal labour.

HypnoBirthing is perfect for home birth as well as hospital birth. A common misconception for homebirthers is that the pain is necessary. Yes, pain is a great communicator when something is wrong, but in a normal labour pain does not have to be present. Through Hypno-Birthing, you may not feel pain, but you will feel the sensation of tightening or pressure. So although you probably won't feel pain, you will know that labour has started, but in sensations that you choose.

Now I know you're probably sceptical as you read this — I felt the same before I discovered HypnoBirthing. Even after teaching my first class, in the back of my mind I was thinking, *I hope this works*". Then one woman from the class called to tell me her story. She had a birth "show" at 9.00 am, felt fine and went about her day. When she went to her 4.00 pm doctor's appointment he checked her cervix and she had already dilated to 6 cm — and she hadn't felt a thing, other than what she described as "strong Braxton Hicks". For all you first-time mums reading this, generally getting from 1 to 6 cm is very long and can be very painful — no doubt your friends have already shared this with you! This woman went on to birth a few hours later and both baby and mum were very happy — it was her doctor who was in shock! I have heard many more stories such as these. This is not a matter of chance, nor were these particular women easier to hypnotise. Rather, they changed their beliefs about birth through a series of classes, which in-clude developing techniques in visualisation and relaxation.

For most mums, birth is that scary day at the end of nine months that you avoid thinking about for eight of those months. Part of you can hardly wait for it because you finally get to meet your little baby, while another part of you wishes you had a time machine, so you could just wake up one day and be handed your baby. Whether we want to admit to it or not, we've already been "hypnotised" to as-sume that the birth will be an ordeal. All we ever hear is how painful it is, on TV, from family and friends. I bet every other preg-nancy/birth book you've read also assumes that birth is intrinsically painful. If this were the case, then it would be so for everyone — and we know it's not. I'm sure you've heard stories of women, maybe even someone you know, who said they didn't even realise they were in labour and gave birth 30 minutes after arriving at the hospi-tal. Remember Laura Shanley's birth story at the beginning of this book? When there is no fear present, labour progresses easily.

HypnoBirthing doesn't involve being in a trance or a sleep or unaware of what is going on. Rather, you'll be able to chat and enjoy birth — totally relaxed, but fully in control. You will always be aware of what is happening to you and around you, and *never* detached from the experience, which is a common misconception especially among medical staff.

Videos of mothers using HypnoBirthing are incredible, showing labouring mothers awake, alert and in good humour as they experience easy and usually quite short births. In fact, these videos are almost strange to watch; we are just not used to seeing birth as such a relaxed experience.

How Hypnosis Works

If you've ever seen hypnosis on TV or gone to see a stage hypnotist you may be a little apprehensive and be afraid that you'll end up barking like a dog each time your mobile rings. Well, it's nothing like that! Try this little experiment. Close your eyes for a moment and take a deep relaxing breath. Notice the sounds around you which you can hear clearly. Then open your eyes. That's what hypnosis feels like. We go in and out of hypnosis all the time. Have you ever been driving somewhere and were thinking about something else and you miss the turn or you get to your destination and don't even remember half of the drive there — that's hypnosis.

There are so many myths around hypnosis that I'll address just the most common ones here. At no time in hypnosis are you "under a spell" or under the control of anyone other than yourself. You are totally in control and fully awake and aware of everything that's going on around you. You can't get "stuck" in hypnosis. In fact, you are in a trance state right now reading this book — you can hear the sounds around you but you choose to focus on what you are reading.

In the US there has been extensive research into the benefits of hypnosis during pregnancy. The most common benefits are fewer complications (mothers aren't stressed), fewer requests for medication (mothers aren't afraid) and have healthier infants (babies are very relaxed).

Without the presence of adrenaline and stress, your body is naturally filled with endorphins — your own epidural and natural pain reliever. When you're afraid, your adrenaline kicks in and your muscles tighten. Try the following little experiment: make a fist with your right hand as tightly as you can and hold it. After a few minutes your hand will start to feel tired and sore. Now relax your hand — see how much more comfortable that is? Mothers who use Hypno-Birthing don't show the usual signs of labour (panic, fear, pain) and sometimes hospital staff don't believe they are in active labour.

It's important to let your caregiver know that you're using HypnoBirthing; most hospitals are supportive, but it's always good to let them know in advance. There are six certified HypnoBirthing educators in Ireland. Contact the HypnoBirthing Institute to find a practitioner near you — see the resources list at the end of the book

I can't emphasise this enough: HypnoBirthing is *not* "pain distraction", and classes do not teach disassociation techniques. Pain is a warning sign that something is wrong and should not be disguised, dissociated from or ignored as is used in traditional hypnotherapy pain "management" techniques.

HYPNOBIRTHING: SARA'S BIRTH STORY

Having watched my tummy expand, having felt movement where there hadn't been any before, and having gone nine months without having any control over which direction my body was expanding, I knew that I was going to have control over one thing: the birth. No fear and knowing I would be able to control my body when it came to the big day — that's what helped me through the whole pregnancy. To add the icing to the cake was the fact that I had achieved the birth that I had planned and prepared for.

Our first baby, Christopher, swam to the surface of the water birthing pool to meet his long-awaited mommy and daddy. He weighed in at a healthy 8lbs 13oz.

The birth was fantastic and the labour very bearable, all due to HypnoBirthing and having Robert there to put me back on the straight and narrow when all I wanted to do was to climb into bed and go asleep and to be woken up when baby was just about there.

I attended the hospital on the day before Christopher's due date for a routine check-up, wondering whether or not they were going to tell me I had another ten days to go until showtime. To my surprise, I was already 2 cm dilated. I couldn't believe it — I hadn't even felt a thing! Needless to say I was sure it was going to happen that night, but he waited until 4.45 am two days later to make any sign of movement. I had had birth shows from the Wednesday evening all the way up to the early hours of Saturday morning. I woke up having only been to bed two hours before — cleaning the house, rechecking bags, eating pineapple — anything to take my mind off the "When will it happen?" question that was going around in my head. I got a pain across my back that was like a strong period paid. I jumped into the shower and got myself ready, then woke Robert and told him it was time to go.

We rang the hospital midwifery-led unit that I was attending, informing them that I was on the way. They had said not to make my way in until I was getting surges that were 10 minutes apart; according to my timing they were coming nearly every five minutes and lasting about 30 seconds. I relaxed my-self and started the HypnoBirthing, thinking of a place that brought back happy memories, imagining how the birth was going to be.

We arrived at the hospital where the midwife led us to the birthing room. I got myself changed and sat on the birthing ball, texting away on my mobile with barely any pains with every surge. The midwife came and did an examination and said that I had reached 5 cm and still had a while to go. We sat in the room laughing and joking, flicking through the television stations. It was very relaxing; lavender oils were burning next to the birthing pool that was waiting to be filled. Throughout the labour I felt warm and drank lots of water, having to make a few trips to the bathroom. When the surges got stronger, I threw up; I knew then that things were progressing further than the midwife had thought.

The pool was filled and I sat into it. The water was lovely; Robert poured it onto my back and talked to me through every surge. We talked about anything and everything, and then put a music CD on to lift the mood. It was still very relaxing; the surges came and went. All that I could think about throughout the labour was that this is how I had imagined it was going to be, and believing that my body was listening to me.

The clock spun on the wall; the time seemed to fly by. Then the urge for baby to birth came. My waters broke around 7.30 am. Christopher's head came out at 8.06 am and finally he emerged fully and swam to the surface at 8.08 am, only 3 hours and 27 minutes from the time I felt the first surge. They had monitored the baby's heart throughout the labour with a doppler and his heart rate had stayed the same. The transition into the world didn't seem to faze him at all. When he arrived he looked up at us, let out a little cry, then lay there quite content. He didn't need to be suctioned at all, and he stayed attached to the placenta until it stopped pulsating.

Throughout the labour Robert talked to me, telling me to breathe the baby down. I got to a stage when the head was coming and I could feel that I was going to tear. It felt to me at that stage as though I had come out of the Hypno-Birthing. Robert tried to get me back but all I could feel was a burning sensation. But once the head had come out it was fine; I relaxed again and knew that everything was over and proud of myself for going through with my plans using hypnobirthing as my form of pain relief.

Unfortunately I ended up having a third-degree tear, which I felt none of after the birth. I could walk fine, but I had to go to surgery where I had to get a spinal block and sedatives. This was my worst nightmare, as I hadn't wanted to receive any medical intervention at all. I had had the birth that we had planned and I had achieved it with no medical intervention and with very little pain. I felt terrible after surgery and was annoyed with myself for tearing — but that's life, and I've got passed that.

I felt groggy and disoriented for four or five days. This was perhaps the feeling I would have felt straight after Christopher was born if I had chosen medication as pain relief.

However I had achieved my ultimate birth experience; I had controlled my labour and birth; HypnoBirthing taught me how. My best friend, who had doubted the hypnobirthing techniques at the start, now thinks it does work; it's all about believing in it and releasing the fear of what others tell you about birth. Robert was in awe of how calm and relaxing the experience was.

I know with the next birth I will do it all over again. Such a wonderful experience, with no fuss or excruciating pain, a natural progression of life, where you are aware of your senses and what's going on around you and that final knowing of what's happening next.

LABOUR IS GOOD FOR BABIES!

Too often we hear these days that babies shouldn't have to "endure" the trauma of childbirth, or that birth is so stressful that an elective caesarean would be much kinder to your little one. In rare cases, this may be true. However, what it boils down to is that the stress of *normal* labour is a good stress ("normal" being a labour that isn't induced or speeded up in any way). As the mother labours, her body produces hormones (endorphins) to help her deal with pain. As she does this, her baby's adrenal glands are stimulated and they begin to produce high levels of adrenaline, or stress hormones. This foetal stress response is designed to help the baby make the transition to life outside the uterus.

The activity of birth helps your baby in the following ways:

- *Helps baby to breathe.* The hormones produced help your newborn keep his lungs expanded. As it keeps the lungs open it helps your baby to clear amniotic fluid from his lungs.

- *Increases blood flow to your baby.* Stress hormones help send more blood to the baby's brain, heart and kidneys.

- *Increases energy supply to the baby.* This is what keeps the baby satisfied until breastmilk comes in.

- *Facilitates bonding.* That alertness your newborn has is directly related to these hormones. A more alert baby draws parents in and he or she is more responsive to parents and others.

- *Increases immunity.* White blood cell numbers are increased as the adrenal hormones are secreted.

Studies have shown that while epidural anaesthesia does not affect the levels of stress hormones, there is a significant difference between babies who are born vaginally versus planned caesarean. If a caesarean does become necessary during labour, even early on, the baby has more adrenaline and adapts to life outside the womb quicker than counterparts born via scheduled caesarean prior to the onset of labour. For this reason, some consultants will delay elective caesarean until after the onset of labour when possible.

© *Robin Elise Weiss and pregnancy.about.com. Reproduced with kind permission*

POSITIONS FOR BIRTH

I have never come across a labouring mother who opted to birth in the traditional (on the back) position voluntarily (unless she's had an epidural). Many will end up back on the bed as a result of staff recommendations. As your baby moves down, it has to navigate the tailbone, which will move out of the way once you are *not* on your back. You're also less likely to get an episiotomy if *you* choose the position you birth in.

The *hands and knees* position can be great for back labour (when your baby's back is lying against yours, also known as OP or posterior presentation). You'll find just rocking your pelvis will be very helpful and can help your baby rotate.

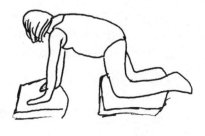

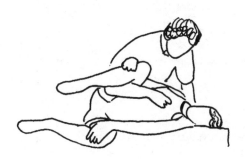

If you've had an epidural or a very long tiring labour, *birthing on your side* with your partner or midwife holding your leg can be helpful. It allows the pelvic bones to expand (but still leaves you vulnerable for an episiotomy).

The *supported squat* is effective but can be tiring for the birth partner. Your birth partner will stand behind you and "hook" you under the arms with his arms. Benefits include an open pelvis and the advantage of gravity. Mum is free to rotate her hips, helping her baby into a good position for birth.

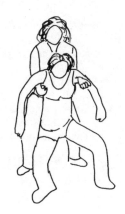

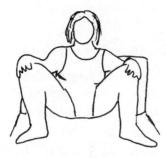

If you have an epidural or just a tiring labour this position is better than the traditional (flat on your back) position.

All Illustrations © Janelle Durham (www.janelledurham.com)

BIRTH PARTNERS! HOW YOU CAN HELP YOUR PARTNER DURING LABOUR

Think "PURRRR":

- *P*osition: Is your partner changing her position regularly and moving about?

- *U*rination: Are you reminding her to go to the bathroom every hour?

- *R*elaxation: Is she as relaxed as possible?

- *R*espiration: Is she breathing even, relaxing breaths and not gasping?

- *R*est: Is she making the most of the break between contractions to rest?

- *R*eassurance: Are you giving her constant encouragement and reassurance?

Tips for your Birth Partner on the big day:

- Remember to eat and drink.

- Wear loose, cool clothing.

- Stay as relaxed as possible.

- Take a break if you need to.

© National Childbirth Trust, www.nctpregnancyandbabycare.com.
Reproduced with kind permission

ROUTINE MEDICAL INTERVENTIONS

FAILURE TO PROGRESS OR FAILURE TO WAIT?

Some Irish hospitals strictly follow active management policies to manage your birth. Once you are admitted you are expected to dilate at approximately 1 cm per hour. (Talk about pressure to perform!) Some women will dilate 1 cm and others may not. As you probably know by now, there's no such thing as a textbook pregnancy or birth. There is some evidence to show that the stress and excitement of arriving at the hospital may trigger adrenaline, which is the body's "fight or flight" response and may cause your dilation to slow down or stop for a time. It is at this crucial time when it is critical that your partner reassures you that you're doing great and helps you to relax. The hormones that are present when you conceived are the same ones you need to help you give birth; for most people, having sex in a brightly lit public area with strangers coming in and out of the room and interrupting them wouldn't exactly set the mood!

What Happens If I Don't Dilate Quickly Enough?

If there are no indications of a medical problem, then patience is your best friend. You can ask *not* to have your labour augmented (speeded up). You can choose not to have your waters broken. You may like to try the more non-invasive method of nipple stimulation or even just a change of position. Nipple stimulation causes a release of oxytocin from the brain, which in turn causes the uterus to contract, and can restart a labour that has slowed down.

No woman is the same, and labour will progress at different rates for everybody — and usually at the right time, all by itself.

When Are Medical Interventions Necessary?

Medical interventions are necessary in a medical emergency but when they are routine (i.e. hospital rules) then they can create problems for the 90 per cent of mothers who have normal births. Episiotomy, forceps delivery, continuous **foetal monitoring, ventouse** delivery and amniotomy are all common medical interventions.

Maybe it's just me, but I don't want anything "routinely" done to me that sounds like lobotomy — such as episiotomy or amniotomy. Following are some of the routine procedures "offered" to mothers in Irish hospitals. The important thing to remember is that if it is done routinely then it definitely isn't supported, in the case of normal births, by current research.

AMNIOTOMY (RUPTURING YOUR MEMBRANES)

Some of you reading this will have had your waters artificially released in hospital. For some women this is not a big deal and labour progresses fine. But there are risks associated with this procedure, and very few benefits. I wonder how many of you have had the following experience: your midwife comes to see you and says, "Let me check you and we'll see how far along we are, shall we?" You look at your hubby, who shrugs his shoulders, and you nod. The midwife roots around for a bit, then announces, "About 3 cm. Now I'm just going to pop your waters so we can see how the baby is doing; you won't feel anything, just a gush of warm water." It's all over in seconds. This scenario is played out in many hospitals throughout Ireland on a daily basis. You have just had a medical intervention performed on you that was not agreed to by informed consent. At no time were the risks and benefits of this procedure explained to you, nor were you given an opportunity to ask about alternatives.

As long as the membranes remain intact, the baby and the cord float inside a water balloon. The fluid protects umbilical cord blood vessels from the pressure of contractions. When you remove the fluid early in labour, that protection is gone and the contractions can impede blood flow, causing foetal distress.

Another risk of early **artificial rupturing of membranes (ARM)** is cord prolapse — that is, the cord descends into the birth canal ahead of the baby. This will most likely result in a section. Routine early amniotomy shortens labour by about an hour but also increases caesarean rates. When data from seven trials in which women were randomly assigned and not assigned to early ARM, the women who had an ARM were 20 per cent more likely to have a section. When left alone, the waters usually release when the cervix has dilated to around 7–8 cm; at this point, your baby has had the benefit of being able to move through the pelvis and get into the best position for birth.

Some hospitals like to rupture membranes routinely to check for meconium (baby's first bowel movement). Meconium in your waters might indicate a stressed baby that needs immediate assistance. Like everything else, nothing is black and white (or brown and green in this case). There are different levels of meconium staining. Your baby could have had a bowel movement weeks ago and is doing fine now and may not warrant a c-section.

Of course there are a few babies who do get distressed, but this is rare in a normal labour. When you take away the amniotic fluid, you can increase the chances of your baby becoming distressed because there is no cushioning between baby and the cord. This is exactly what the hospital was trying to avoid in the first place. Like most routine procedures, it makes no sense and the current research confirms this. The easiest way to avoid these routine procedures is to stay home as long as possible and educate yourself on the risks of each intervention you are "offered".

Procedure	Artificial rupture of the bag of waters (Amniotomy)
What is it?	Breaking the amniotic sac surrounding the baby with an amniohook
Who needs it?	When there are other signs of distress there may be a need to see the colour of the amniotic fluid
Who doesn't need it?	Most pregnant women
Risks	1. Sets "time clock" running for need to deliver your baby 2. Infection 3. Prolapse of umbilical cord if done too early 4. Decrease in pH of newborns with early amniotomy 5. Umbilical cord compression (increase of foetal distress)
Benefit	Small decrease in labour time

Source: Janelle Durham (www.janelledurham.com)

No Eating and Drinking in Labour

Routine withholding of food and drink from all mothers is an outdated and dangerous policy. Research suggests that mothers who are prohibited from eating and drinking at will tend to tire easily in labour and are more likely to end up with a caesarean.

The main reason given for such a policy is that, if general anaesthesia is required, it reduces the risk of aspiration. However, this has been shown to be an issue with the anaesthetist's skill level and not with the fact that the mother has eaten during labour. Even a mother who has fasted will have gastric fluid in her stomach which would be just as damaging and more acidic.

Procedure	Policy of NPO (Non Per Os — Latin for Nil by Mouth)
What is it?	Mother is allowed nothing by mouth
Who needs it?	Women who are very ill (a specific medical indication)
Who doesn't need it?	Pregnant women who are not ill
Risks	1. Lack of energy to do the work of labour 2. Dehydration 3. Poor foetal heart rate tracing due to maternal dehydration
Benefit	Reduces the risk of aspiration under general anaesthetic (debatable).

Source: Janelle Durham (www.janelledurham.com)

EPIDURAL

The epidural is the most common way of managing pain in labour (see pages 81–82). The epidural works by injecting a pain medication near particular nerves in the back, blocking these nerves from transmitting pain sensations to the brain. The effect of the epidural is localised to your abdomen, lower back and legs. The anaesthetist will place a sterile drape over your back, and wipe it with an antiseptic solution. You may feel a sting from the injection to freeze the area of your lower back where the epidural needle is being placed. Between contractions, you should only feel pressure as the epidural needle passes between two vertebrae to the epidural space. A thin plastic tube is passed through the needle and the needle is then removed. The remaining flexible tube is taped to your back.

A new development in Irish maternity care is a patient-controlled pump, so that you can receive medication when you need it; this is not available in every hospital.

Is it the Right Choice for You?

Most women who receive an epidural appreciate the respite from pain; they do, however, acknowledge that there are trade-offs involved. You may experience shaking, itchiness and nausea. You'll also need continuous monitoring, an IV and a catheter to drain your urine. A few women get incomplete pain relief or find that it just doesn't work.

The epidural affects your experience of labour, and not always positively. The epidural limits a woman's ability to use a variety of positions to help the baby rotate and descend into the pelvis.

The epidural has many potential side effects — see table below. Did you ever wonder why you can't have an epidural at a home birth? It's because the potential side effects are so risky they couldn't be managed at home.

A rare side effect of the epidural is a severe headache, caused by the epidural needle being inserted too far: instead of stopping in the epidural space, the needle punctures the membrane that surrounds the spinal cord. Sometimes, an injection to "patch" the spot that was pierced by the epidural needle is used to relieve a very bad headache.

Remember that the epidural is only one pain-relieving technique. You will need others to get you through early labour and possibly later labour as well. Even with an epidural, you may experience small windows of pain or a return of pain when it is time to push your baby out. Now is the time to learn and rehearse coping skills. Many women find techniques and good support are all they need to cope with contractions right through to the birth (see pages 83–96). But for those who want more pain relief, or who are unfortunate enough to experience unusually long or complicated labours, the epidural can be a wonderful option.

Birth partners: remember that your job is not over just because mum is physically feeling more comfortable after an epidural. Your partner still needs lots of emotional support and encouragement during this time.

Procedure	Epidural anaesthesia
What is it?	Regional anaesthesia of lower two-thirds of body
Who needs it?	Women who do not have access to comfort measures and are not able to tolerate or don't want to tolerate the pain of labour; some women with high blood pressure.
Who doesn't need it?	Women with continuous support and access to a wide variety of comfort measures and maternal positions; women with blood-clotting problems.
Risks	1. Decrease in maternal blood pressure 2. Decrease in foetal heart rate 3. Lack of variability in foetal heart rate 4. Mother often needs a catheter (can't feel a full bladder) 5. Increase in chance for urinary infection 6. Itching 7. Prolonged labour 8. Increase in need for instrumental delivery via forceps or vacuum aspiration 9. Reported increase (in some studies) of caesarean section (two to fourfold), especially in first-time mothers 10. Increase in need for episiotomy 11. Headache 12. Respiratory arrest or paralysis in rare cases 13. Increase in labour interventions 14. Infection 15. Ineffective pain relief 16. Increase in maternal temperature 17. Breastfeeding difficulties. (babies may be sleepy and have no interest in the breast) 18. Mobility is affected for some time after the birth.
Benefit	Pain relief when other comfort measures are ineffective or when a caesarean section is needed.

Source: Janelle Durham (www.janelledurham.com)

Continuous Foetal Monitoring

Listening to the baby's heart has been used for many years to gain a sense of how the baby is doing during labour. Initially it was thought that this continuous monitoring would reduce incidents of brain damage to babies because distress could be picked up quickly. Not so. Continuous foetal monitoring was not the silver bullet it was expected to be. Midwives and doctors began to spend more time "mothering the machine" instead of mothering the mother.

There are a variety of ways that you can check your baby's heart rate — **fetoscope** (a modified stethoscope), handheld **doppler** unit and the **electronic foetal monitor (EFM)**. The fetoscope and handheld doppler are used for "intermittent" monitoring — the heart rate is measured over a short period of time (e.g. during a contraction). The EFM can be used either intermittently or continuously and creates a permanent record of the baby's heart rate on paper. EFM can be done externally, by using two sensors strapped to the mother's belly (one measures uterine contractions and the other measures the heart rate via doppler). EFM can also be done internally, via a pressure catheter inserted in the uterus to detect contractions and a small electrode that is "clipped" into the baby's scalp, to detect the heart rate. Internal monitoring requires that the bag of waters or membranes are ruptured. EFM provides beat-to-beat view of the baby's heart tones, in relationship to mother's contractions. This is a benefit for the high-risk mother, but of questionable benefit to the low risk mother. Continuous external monitoring uses ultrasound; leaves room for mechanical error, which may cause incorrect interpretation, unnecessary interventions etc.; your movement is limited (when in use), which may slow labour; and may switch attention from the mother to the machine. Continuous electronic monitoring is not recommended for normal birth. Using a fetoscope or doppler intermittently is just as effective in checking your baby's well-being.

Procedure	Continuous electronic foetal monitoring
What is it?	Continuous electronic tracing of foetal heart rate
Who needs it?	A foetus with intrauterine growth retardation or an ill foetus or a baby considered high risk.
Who doesn't need it?	Normal babies, although checking the foetal heart tones periodically is as effective and complies with The American College of Obstetricians and Gynaecologists (ACOG) standards
Risks	1. Increases rate of caesarean section unnecessarily 2. Increases in false diagnosis of foetal distress
Benefit	Constant surveillance of an ill baby

Source: Janelle Durham (www.janelledurham.com)

EPISIOTOMY

Of all the squeamish discussions about birth experiences, probably nothing makes you cringe and cross your legs quicker than when talk about labour turns to the big E — no, not the epidural, but the episiotomy.

More and more women in Ireland are questioning a once-routine procedure that involves enlarging the opening of the birth canal as the baby's head crowns. Your doctor or midwife makes an incision in the perineum (the tissue between the vagina and anus). Some hospitals continue this outdated procedure despite significant studies that show routine episiotomies cause more harm than good.

First a simple demonstration: if you hold a piece of cloth at two corners and attempt to tear it by pulling at the two ends, it's very difficult to rip. However, if you make a small snip in the centre, and pull the corners the cloth rips easily with no resistance.

According to www.maternitywise.org, those who support the practice claim that episiotomies have the following benefits:

- Speed up the birth

- Prevent tearing
- Protect against incontinence
- Protect against **pelvic floor** relaxation
- Heal easier than tears.

The following have been reported as side effects of the episiotomy:

- Infection
- Increased pain
- Increase in third and fourth degree vaginal lacerations (euphemistically called extensions)
- Longer healing times
- Increased discomfort when intercourse is resumed.

Routine episiotomy (as opposed to episiotomy for an emergency situation such as foetal distress) is a typical example of an obstetrical procedure that still exists despite a total lack of evidence for it and a considerable body of evidence against it. So how can you avoid an unnecessary episiotomy? Some preventative measures that www.maternitywise.org recommend are:

- Choose a doctor who doesn't do routine episiotomies. Ask your caregiver how often he/she finds it necessary to do episiotomies.
- Good nutrition.
- Do your Kegels (exercise for your pelvic floor muscles).
- Prenatal perineal massage.
- Slow controlled pushing instead of directed pushing by doctors and midwives — only push when you feel the urge (see below).
- Birth off the bed, not on your back.

Remember, as with any medical procedure, there are always circumstances where episiotomy is a valid and necessary option. The only time most caregivers would agree that an episiotomy is appropriate is when the baby is close to being born and an urgent problem develops.

EPISIOTOMY: MYTHS AND REALITIES

When examined in scientific studies, none of the reasons given for the common or routine use of episiotomy hold up, including:

- *Woman is a first-time mother*: Studies that attempt to restrict episiotomy do not find that having a first baby is, in and of itself, a reason for episiotomy (in some Irish hospitals, at least a quarter of first-time mothers are surgically cut).

- *Caregiver believes a tear is about to occur*: Performing an episiotomy for this reason has not been shown to have a protective effect and may be counter-productive.

- *Belief that episiotomy prevents pelvic floor weakness*: Women are just as likely to have weak pelvic floors or urinary incontinence in the early months after childbirth with or without an episiotomy — caused by the pregnancy, not necessarily the birth. Women with no episiotomy and no or only a tiny tear at birth (intact perineum) have the strongest pelvic floors, while women with tears into the anal muscle have the weakest pelvic floors. Women with spontaneous tears do just as well as, or better than, women with episiotomies.

- *Belief that episiotomy is easier to repair (to stitch closed) than a tear*: No research supports this claim. Certainly the tear that occurs when a midline episiotomy extends into the anal muscle is more difficult to repair than a small tear. With optimal care, many women will need no more than a few stitches or no stitches at all.

- *Belief that episiotomy heals better*: An episiotomy of either type is more likely to have delayed healing or to become infected in comparison with no episiotomy. A mediolateral episiotomy is more likely to scar and heal pulled to one side compared with the tears that may occur with no episiotomy.

© *www.maternitywise.org. Reproduced with kind permission.*

Procedure	Episiotomy
What is it?	Surgical incision in the perineal muscles and tissue.
Who needs it?	Women whose babies must be delivered immediately due to low heart tones.
Who doesn't need it?	Most women in childbirth.
Risks	1. Increase in third- and fourth-degree lacerations involving the rectal sphincter 2. Postoperative pain 3. Sexual dysfunction due to long-term perineal pain 4. Infection.
Benefit	Minimal decrease in length of second-stage labour and speeds delivery in a real emergency

Source: *Janelle Durham (www.janelledurham.com)*

IMMEDIATE CORD CLAMPING

According to the WHO: "Late **clamping** (or not clamping at all) is the physiological way of treating the cord, and early clamping is an intervention that needs justification . . . in normal birth there should be a valid reason to interfere with the natural procedure." When your baby has been born, ideally the cord should be allowed to stop pulsating before being cut or clamped. This ensures that your baby receives all the blood intended for him.

Procedure	Immediate Cord Clamping
What is it?	Cord is clamped and cut within minutes of your baby being born.
Who needs it?	Only women having a managed third stage who have had syntometrine (synthetic oxytocin) to expel the placenta.
Who doesn't need it?	Most pregnant women.
Risks	1. Deprives your baby of oxygen; if your baby is having breathing difficulties immediately after birth and the cord is still pulsating, it makes sense to keep the cord intact so the baby has two sources of oxygen as he adjusts to breathing outside the womb. 2. Deprives your baby of nutrients through placental blood supply 3. Reduces your baby's total blood volume by approx one-third.

Source: Janelle Durham (www.janelledurham.com)

OTHER INTERVENTIONS

Sometimes if your caregiver suspects your baby is in distress or if you've had a long labour and are just too exhausted to push, your doctor may need to use a forceps or vacuum to deliver your baby. You're more likely to need some help with the last few pushes if you've had an epidural. The epidural relaxes the pelvic floor, so it doesn't have the resistance that your baby needs to rotate into a good birth position and seems "stuck".

Forceps

Forceps look like metal salad tongs. It comes in two pieces that your doctor will insert into your vagina (you'll never quite look at salad tongs the same way again) and place around the sides of your baby's head. There is a mechanism to fix the forceps once they have been correctly placed so that they don't come apart. Your midwife will probably put her hand on your bump and watch the monitor to see when there is another contraction coming. You'll then be instructed to bear down and push hard with your next contraction as the doctor pulls. You'll most likely be given an episiotomy.

In general babies born with forceps are fine but can sustain minor bruising to the head and face, so don't be alarmed.

Ventouse

The ventouse is a suction cap made of silicone plastic. It fits onto the baby's head rather like a little cap. Once the cap has been positioned, air is sucked out of it by means of a vacuum device (like a bicycle pump). The doctor then pulls as the mother pushes; just like with the forceps, often a midwife will also be pushing on your bump to move your baby down the birth canal.

Some babies can be quite bruised after a ventouse delivery in the form of a blood blister around the area of the vacuum cap and may develop some jaundice from it. After a long labour your baby may appear quite cone-headed and the blister may accentuate that, but it's usually superficial and doesn't affect your baby's brain. The swelling usually goes down after a few days.

Research suggests that a ventouse delivery is better for mum and baby as there appears to be less damage to the mother's pelvic floor and it is gentler than a forceps delivery. Assisted deliveries can be scary for you, your partner and your baby, so the best advice is to avoid interventions that can directly or indirectly increase your chances of needing them (amniotomy, epidural, birthing on your back).

Directed/Coached Pushing

Another less-known "intervention" which is coming under scrutiny is **directed or coached pushing** (also known as the **valsalva** or purple pushing). Many researchers now suggest that, once the second stage is reached, a period of rest should be allowed before any vigorous pushing in order to allow the head to descend and rotate slowly, allowing gentle stretching of the tissues and conserving energy. Directed pushing only reduces the birthing time by a few minutes. In an undisturbed natural birth, there is a phenomenon called the **foetal ejection reflex** — in other words, without any active pushing, your body will automatically push the baby out in an uncontrollable reflex action.

From experience, it would appear that the majority of caregivers encourage directed pushing with breath-holding in the second stage (pushing stage) of labour to speed things up. It's unclear why this is so common, most likely because it's just how the hospital has done things for a long time. However, there is now evidence to indicate that encouraged, strenuous pushing may not be the most appropriate means of managing this part of labour and mothers should be encouraged to do what feels right for them.

- *Risks for your Baby*: Directed pushing causes a rise in blood pressure, followed by a rapid fall which is only relieved on release of the breath. Several studies have found this to be problematic, causing lack of oxygen to the placenta and baby. Conversely, when pushing was spontaneous (only pushing when you feel the urge or, if you have an epidural, only when the monitor shows a contraction starting), using only the abdominal muscles and with slow exhalation, the baby's heart rate tended to either be maintained at baseline levels or, if decelerations occurred, recovered more quickly.

- *Risks for Mothers*: Directed pushing can cause blood pressure to drop, causing dizziness and a strain on the heart. There is also risk of maternal exhaustion. Directed pushing is also associated with more perineal trauma (those nasty tears) and more postpartum perineal and vaginal pain than does delayed, spontaneous pushing. You also may end up with broken veins on your face and bloodshot eyes . . . not exactly the first thing you want your newborn seeing! And wouldn't it be nice for your baby to be born into a room where the first voice he hears is your voice, or at least quiet voices, rather than three people saying *PUUUSH*?

CASCADE OF INTERVENTION

Obstetric interventions can be life-saving procedures for women and babies. Technological advances in proven surgical techniques and better anaesthetics have ensured that the 20 per cent of women who need this kind of help receive the best possible care.

Once the natural process of labour and birth has been disturbed, especially if there is no actual medical emergency, there is a significant risk that the unwelcome side effects of the treatment will make further intervention necessary to remedy the problem. This phenomenon is known as the cascade of intervention and is illustrated in the diagram below. It's like the domino effect: once it's started, it has a knock-on effect in your labour and more interventions become necessary.

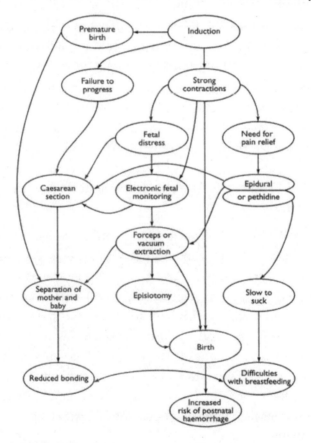

Source: © Birth International

MULTIPLE BIRTHS

WHAT IF IT'S TWINS?

The diagnosis of twins can feel like an out-of-body experience for many. You may have suspected that something was up because you've never felt so sick in your life (caused by a sudden increase in hormones), but when you're given the news that there are two or even three heartbeats you may feel like you've just entered the twilight zone. Most consultants consider twin pregnancies high risk, which does not imply that the birth will be a normal, full-term one, but it does mean that the hospital will monitor you more closely. About half of all multiple pregnancies result in premature births (i.e. before week 37), but unless and until that happens to you, focus on being in the half that go the full term.

You will undoubtedly have to see your consultant or midwife more often — probably weekly by the sixth month — and your own health and the babies' progress will be very closely monitored.

POSSIBLE COMPLICATIONS

Aside from the chance that your babies will be born prematurely, the most common problems include:

- You're going to feel HUGE. Get lots of rest and get help from family and friends. If you've already had a baby, then think of the way you felt when you were nine months' pregnant . . . then back that up to about seven months . . . in other words, two extra months of fat fingers, swollen ankles and sore muscles.

- **Pre-eclampsia** develops in about 10 to 20 per cent of women carrying twins

- **Placental abruption** is also more common for multiple births. Thankfully this is a very rare complication.

- Foetal growth restriction, when one or both twins isn't growing at the proper rate, may cause the babies to be born prematurely or at a low birth weight. About half of pregnancies with more than one baby have this problem.

- Twin–twin transfusion syndrome is another rare but serious complication in identical twins. One baby gets too much blood and the other too little. Early detection is critical for twin to twin syndrome.

What Happens if I have one of these Complications?

Once you get to about 36 weeks, the risk of delivering a premature or low-birthweight baby decreases significantly. Before this, any complications may require medications, hospitalisation or bedrest. Educate yourself about the more common risks and complications of a twin pregnancy, while trying not to obsess about the things that can go wrong. There are lots of twin support groups that you can connect with to help you focus on the positives. Familiarise yourself with the warning signs of pre-term labour (e.g. waters breaking before 37 weeks or persistent contractions). Make sure you are eating well and staying well hydrated.

What Happens if I'm Put on Bedrest?

If you go into labour early some caregivers will recommend **bedrest**, depending on their policies, even though no research has proven that bedrest will prevent a pre-term birth.

You're may be reading this thinking, *"Wouldn't bedrest be soooo nice . . . start my maternity leave early . . . no more dragging myself out of bed on those dark January mornings . . . I can just roll over and go back to sleep."* Bedrest can be excruciatingly boring. Sure, a few days in bed can sometimes be just what the doctor ordered, pregnant or not — but two months of it? Be careful what you wish for.

If you are put on bedrest, find out exactly what that means, because the definition can vary from slightly curtailing your activity to literally not getting out of bed for any reason — and everything in between. Bedrest means something different for every woman depending on what the problem is. The following list from Sidelines, a US-based support group for mums on bed rest, can help you nail down the specifics:

- How long will I need to be on bedrest?
- Can I get up to use the bathroom?
- What position should I rest in?
- Can I still do things around the house like washing and cooking?
- Can I drive at all?
- Can I work at home in bed with a laptop?
- Can I lift anything?
- How often is it safe to stand?
- What about caring for my other children? What can — and what can't — I do?
- Are there any exercises I can do while on bedrest?
- If I'm prescribed tocolytics (a medication that helps reduce pre-term contractions), what do I need to know about it? Are there any side effects?

For tips on surviving bedrest, contact Sidelines.org.

When Things Are Not Going to Plan

Big Baby Syndrome

Having a "big" baby is a major fear of women facing childbirth. Babies are bigger and healthier these days, but the majority of mums are also healthier too. Years ago when Irish mothers barely had enough decent nutritious food to eat, a diagnosis of a big baby would be a huge relief, simply because big babies were usually a sign of healthy babies. You don't have to look very far these days to hear very healthy women talking about how their baby has been deemed "big" and they are probably going to have a caesarean because they aren't big enough to give birth. When did we buy into the myth that we are destined to be failures at birth? Other mammals don't seem to have these problems.

CPD? Don't Panic!

A diagnosis of **CPD (cephalopelvic disproportion)** means the baby's head is thought to be too large to pass through the woman's pelvis. In the eighteenth and nineteenth centuries, poor nutrition, rickets and illnesses such as polio caused pelvic anomalies, which resulted in loss of life during childbirth. Indeed initially CPD was the most common reason for carrying out a caesarean. In modern times, however, true CPD is rare, since our general standard of living is so much higher and true CPD is more likely to be caused by pelvic fracture due to road traffic accidents or congenital abnormalities (see page 126).

Often CPD is implied rather than diagnosed. In cases where labour has failed to progress (or your consultant has "failed to wait") or the baby has become distressed, medical staff commonly assume that this is due to physical inadequacies in the mother rather than looking towards circumstances of the mother's care. These problems frequently occur when CPD is not suspected and there are many other causes such as fear and uncertainty, difficulty adjusting to a medical environment, lack of emotional support and non-continuity of carer.

CPD is also sometimes suspected when the baby's head fails to engage, although both this and failure to progress have proved unreliable indicators.

A woman's degree of motivation to achieve a vaginal delivery along with the level of support she receives are likely to be more influential on the outcome than her pelvic measurements. Even in undisputed cases of CPD, it should still be possible for a mother to go into labour without compromising the safety of her baby. In fact, a period of labour prior to caesarean section is believed to reduce the occurrence of respiratory distress and can therefore be beneficial for the baby.

In any case, CPD is difficult to diagnose accurately, since there are no less than four variables that cannot be measured:

- The pelvis is not a fixed, solid structure. During pregnancy and labour, the hormone relaxin softens the ligaments that join the pelvic bones, allowing the pelvis to give and expand. The degree of pelvic expansion achieved will vary from woman to woman and from pregnancy to pregnancy.

- Babies' heads are made up of separate bones, which move relative to each other, allowing the baby's head to "mould" and reduce its diameter during passage down the birth canal. No one can predict the capacity of an individual baby's head to mould and, as this is a feature of the normal birth process, should not adversely affect the health and well-being of the baby.

- The position that a woman adopts during labour and delivery makes a significant difference to pelvic dimensions. Squatting, for example, can increase pelvic measurements by up to 30 per cent. One of the most common positions in which women give birth, that of being semi-reclined, where the mother's weight is on her coccyx (tail bone), restricts movement of the coccyx, which can severely compromise a below-average pelvis.

- The position of the baby can be crucial, and whether its head is well flexed or tilted can mean the difference between an easy delivery and delivery being impossible.

When a diagnosis of CPD has been made, many people still believe that this constitutes a reason for elective repeat caesarean section in future pregnancies, despite the wealth of evidence to the contrary. Indeed, there have been many documented cases where women have been diagnosed as having CPD and then gone on to deliver vaginally a larger infant than the one that was delivered surgically.

Some women will be able to accept a diagnosis of CPD, perhaps even preferring the caesarean way of birth, whereas others will want to be able to come to their own independent conclusions, and some of these may wish to labour again under more conducive circumstances, to have the chance to give labour their "best shot".

© www.caesarean.org. Reproduced with kind permission.

WHAT IF MY BABY IS BREECH?

If you've just been told that your baby is breech (i.e. your baby's legs or backside are coming first instead of his head), take a deep breath, relax and let's talk about it. If you are still less than 37 weeks pregnant, then the good news is that your baby will most likely turn before labour without you doing anything!

If you are 37 weeks or more, you still have choices. Recent research concluded that caesarean section was the preferred birth option, but this study has been heavily criticised and now has consultants all over the world rethinking their approach to breech births. In Ireland most breech births are via caesarean section but some doctors will help you birth a breech baby.

BREECH BIRTH: WHAT ARE YOUR OPTIONS?

If you decide to opt for a caesarean birth, it is advisable to wait until labour begins before the surgery is performed, as this will eliminate the risk of prematurity and give the baby the benefits of the labour contractions, which are important to get your baby's lungs ready to breathe on their own.

Shop around for a caregiver if your baby is breech and you want a vaginal birth. In countries and hospitals where vaginal breech births are a common occurrence, the outcomes for mums and babies are good. There is also evidence that hypnosis can be very successful for turning a breech baby and in one study hypnosis proved to be more successful than manually turning the baby by **ECV (External Cephalic Version)** (see below).

External Cephalic Version

Research indicates that manually manipulating the baby into a better position is often successful for turning breech babies if done around 38–39 weeks. You will need to find a caregiver skilled in this procedure, and you will need to take a drug to relax the muscles of the uterus while it is being done. As there is always a very slight risk that the cord will become entangled or the placenta start to separate as the baby is turned, external cephalic version should always be done in a hospital, where a caesarean section is available in the unlikely event of such an emergency.

ECV is not pleasant. It's not exactly a gentle manipulation; some force is required by your consultant and probably a midwife. Even after an ECV, some babies will still flip back to a breech position, although it's less likely when done at 38 weeks due to the size of the baby.

If, after trying everything, the baby does not move into a head-down position, there may be a good reason why he prefers to remain in the breech position; perhaps the placenta is positioned low down, limiting the space for the baby's head in the lower part of the uterus, or the uterus itself is shaped unusually and is restricting his movements. If the baby does not turn easily, then it must be assumed that he needs to stay where he is (babies are smarter than we think).

"Moxa"

A very successful "do it yourself" technique with a proven high success rate is to use locally applied heat treatment.

The heat from burning moxa sticks — called **"moxibustion"** — can be used to stimulate the baby's movements and encourage it to turn. These sticks, shaped like cigars, are available from herbalists, Chinese medicine stockists and some acupuncturists (who use moxa sticks for other purposes) and they contain tightly rolled dried leaves of the mugwort plant. They are very inexpensive and two sticks will be needed — they can be used several times.

A randomised controlled trial indicates that approximately 70 per cent of breech babies will turn using this method.

© Andrea Robertson and Birth International, www.birthinternational.com.
Reproduced with kind permission

Hypnosis

Although hypnosis is usually associated with giving up cigarettes or losing weight, one of the most interesting new areas of study is the effect it has on babies in a breech presentation in utero. Hypnosis is very effective in changing the position of a breech baby, persuading it to turn, often within minutes of the session. A study on breech babies turned with hypnosis, also showed that these babies stayed in the proper position, where babies turned manually often returned to the breech position.

This ability for the baby to be influenced by the mother's thoughts and suggestions give us even more evidence that we are in communication with our babies throughout our pregnancies.

Acupuncture is another option worth trying.

WHAT IF MY BABY IS IN THE POSTERIOR POSITION?

If you are told your baby is "posterior", this means he is facing your tummy instead of your backside; i.e. your baby's back is against yours. Mothers of babies in the "posterior" position can (but not always) end up with long and painful "back" labours as the baby usually has to turn all the way round to facing the back in order to be born. If you're having back labour, then the last place you will want to be is on your back. You'll instinctively get on all fours or into a position that helps your baby rotate into a better position.

You may be able to reduce the likelihood of a posterior presentation by being aware of your posture during pregnancy. There are also "tricks" for turning posterior babies, if yours seems stubborn. These are not evidence based — just recommendations from mothers who had posterior births on what worked for them.

TIPS FOR TURNING A POSTERIOR BABY BEFORE LABOUR

Avoid positions that encourage your baby to face your tummy. The main culprits are said to be lolling back in armchairs, sitting in car seats where you are leaning back, or anything where your knees are higher than your pelvis.

- The best way to do this is to spend lots of time kneeling upright, or sitting upright, or on hands and knees. When you sit on a chair, make sure your knees are lower than your pelvis, and your trunk should be tilted slightly forwards.

- Watch TV while kneeling on the floor, over a beanbag or cushions, or sit on a dining chair. Try sitting on a dining chair facing (leaning on) the back as well.

- Use yoga positions while resting, reading or watching TV — for example, tailor pose (sitting with your back upright and soles of the feet together, knees out to the sides)

- Sit on a wedge cushion in the car, so that your pelvis is tilted forwards. Keep the seat back upright.

- Don't cross your legs! This reduces the space at the front of the pelvis, and opens it up at the back. For good positioning, the baby needs to have lots of space at the *front*.

- Don't put your feet up! Lying back with your feet up encourages posterior presentation.

- Sleep on your side, not on your back.

- Avoid deep squatting, which opens up the pelvis and encourages the baby to move down, until you know he/she is the right way round. Jean Sutton recommends squatting on a low stool instead, and keeping your spine upright, not leaning forwards.

- Swimming with your belly downwards is said to be very good for positioning babies — not backstroke, but lots of breaststroke and front crawl. Breaststroke in particular is thought to help with good positioning, because all those leg movements help open your pelvis and settle the baby downwards.

- A birth ball can encourage good positioning, both before and during labour.

- Various exercises done on all fours can help, e.g. wiggling your hips from side to side, or arching your back like a cat, followed by dropping the spine down. This is described in more detail in an article on www.wellmother.org — "Exercise for relieving backache" by Suzanne Yates.

CAESAREAN SECTION

PLEASE READ ME!

Don't skip this chapter and assume it won't happen to you. Ireland and most of the Western world has a serious problem with caesarean rates that continue to climb, despite the fact that the vast majority of these women and babies are generally in good health. The chances are that, at a minimum, one in every four women reading these pages today will end up with an unplanned or emergency **caesarean section**. It is human nature to think that it won't happen to you, so please don't skip this chapter.

According to the Report of Perinatal Statistics for 2002, 22.4 per cent of all births in Ireland in 2002 were by caesarean section. Despite government initiatives to reduce the number of caesareans, the number of babies being delivered surgically has doubled, or even tripled, at many maternity units during the past ten years.

Reasons cited for the rise include better detection of foetal distress, more older women having babies, an increased tendency among patients to resort to litigation, doctors wanting to speed up births, patients' preference and — most unbelievably — babies growing too big in utero.

WHEN IS IT NECESSARY?

Much depends on whether your consultant (or midwife) follows a policy of active management or expectant management; an active management policy is more likely result in a caesarean.

Caesareans will almost certainly be performed in the following cases:

- *Transverse lie*: Your baby is lying sideways.

• *True CPD*: True **cephalopelvic disproportion (CPD)** occurs when a baby's head or body is too large to fit through the mother's pelvis. True CPD is very rare, but many cases of "failure to progress" labour are given this diagnosis. When an *accurate* diagnosis of CPD has been made, the safest type of delivery for mother and baby is a caesarean delivery. The problem is, true CPD cannot be diagnosed until during labour.

 • *Placenta previa*: When the placenta is blocking the cervical opening. A complete **placenta previa** (i.e. when the placenta is *completely* blocking the opening) in late pregnancy would automatically mean a c-section and maybe even a few weeks of bedrest beforehand. It's quite normal to have some kind of previa mid-pregnancy, but the placenta usually moves up as the uterus grows. In other words, it will normally self correct — no need for you to do anything.

 • *Prolapsed cord* (i.e. when the cord comes out before your baby) in the first stage of labour.

Other reasons given for caesreans (usually by consultants with an active management philosophy), but which may not be absolutely necessary include:

• *Relative CPD*: The baby is poorly positioned for delivery, such as a posterior baby (baby is lying with its back to your back). In order to avoid a caesarean, there are ways to help your baby get into the best position for birth (see pages 123–124). Also, avoiding artificial rupture of membranes is important so the baby can make its way through the pelvis with the cushioning of the amniotic fluid.

• *Foetal Distress*: This is an indicator that your baby may not be doing well in labour. Foetal distress is very subjective; in Ireland, some consultants will take a sample of blood from your baby's scalp, if they suspect foetal distress, to see if your baby is truly being deprived of oxygen. Sometimes just changing position can help. Foetal distress is more common in labours that are induced or augmented with syntocinon.

- **Dystocia** *of Labour (Failure to Progress)*: This basically means that your time is up according to the active management school of thinking; with an expectant management consultant, as long as mum and baby are doing well the labour would continue.

- *Maternal Exhaustion*: This occurs when a woman has had an unusually long labour and is too tired to push.

What Normally Happens During a Caesarean?

If you don't have an epidural already you'll be taken to theatre where an anaesthetist will inject the epidural into your back. You may have some stinging while the area of your back is numbed so the epidural or spinal injection can be inserted but this is usually momentary. You may have some shivering which can result both from the anaesthesia and stress. You will be given a catheter to drain your urine; this is done after the epidural has taken effect, so you won't feel anything. These days it's quite normal for partners to be present during a caesarean, provided you have an epidural and don't need a general anaesthetic, which is rare. Check hospital policy on this.

You will be put on an IV containing fluid and, possibly, drugs. You will probably also be put on oxygen. However, if the epidural doesn't work, you'll be knocked out with a general anaesthetic. If you are just under local anaesthetic, a little "curtain" will be hung below your neck so you don't have to look at the surgery. Sometimes it is possible to see the surgery in the mirrored overhead lights. If you can see anything, try to focus on something else. Birth partners: help keep mum positive and focus on the fact that you'll be meeting your little one soon.

Your pubic hair is shaved and an incision is made, horizontally, just above the pubic bone. You'll probably hear lots of odd noises like the suction machine. Birth partners: stay as calm as you can and focus on your partner's face, especially if blood makes you queasy.

You may feel intense pulling and tugging to dislodge the baby's head from the pelvis. If your baby is in the head-down position (**vertex**), your baby is pulled by the neck backwards out of the pelvis (sometimes with forceps) and then by the head through the incision in the uterus (it's quite small). The baby's nose and mouth are then suctioned to remove any amniotic fluid, mucous and/or meconium from the airway. The remainder of the baby's body is pulled from your uterus through the incision, taking care not to tear the uterine or abdominal incision wider.

Your baby will be checked over while you are being stitched. The umbilical cord is clamped and cut immediately and your baby will be dried off and weighed. Syntocinon/Pitocin is immediately injected into the mother's IV to begin contractions of the uterus to aid in the removal of the placenta. The placenta is removed and examined to ensure all pieces are intact. . . . One set of stitches is made in the wall of the uterus, then a second layer of stitches in the outer lining. . . . The abdominal cavity is washed out with water to flush out any bacteria (to prevent infection) and check for bleeding. Your abdomen is then stitched and you are then moved to the recovery area. From the time of the epidural, you should see your baby in about 10 minutes, but the stitching up takes an additional 30–40 minutes.

Within 24 hours, the urine catheter is removed and you are allowed to stand and perhaps walk to the bathroom or shower, but you probably won't want to. Within five days you'll be discharged, with a check of the incision in two weeks. If you think the scar may be infected you'll need antibiotics. Incision pain may occur constantly or intermittently for up to a year. (*Source:* International Caesarean Network.)

Breastfeeding is not impossible after a caesarean but it is much more difficult. Try to get your baby on the breast as soon as you get to recovery, provided your baby is doing OK. Some hospitals insist on taking the baby to the nursery after a caesarean birth but you can request that your baby stay with you in recovery if he is doing well. Ask to see a **lactation consultant**. Side-lying to breastfeed will make initial breastfeeding easier. Probably the hardest part of breastfeeding after a caesarean is just getting out of bed to get your baby. Ask the midwife to bring your baby to you as often as you need to nurse him or have someone stay with you as much as possible during the first few days at the hospital to help pass the baby to you. Surgery can affect how quickly your milk comes in too, so don't be surprised if your milk takes a little longer to come in after a caesarean. (It's usually two or three days for a normal birth.)

RISKS OF CAESAREAN SECTION

Risks for the mother include the following:

- *Infection*: The uterus or nearby pelvic organs such as the bladder or kidneys can become infected.

- *Increased blood loss*: Blood loss on average is about twice as much with caesarean birth as with vaginal birth. However, blood transfusions are rarely needed during a caesarean.

- *Decreased bowel function*: The bowel sometimes slows down for several days after surgery, resulting in distention, bloating and discomfort.

- *Respiratory complications*: General anaesthesia can sometimes lead to pneumonia (general anaesthesia use is rare for a caesarean)

- *Longer hospital stay and recovery time*: Five days in the hospital is the common length of stay, whereas it is less than one to three days for a vaginal birth.

- *Reactions to anaesthesia*: The mother's health could be endangered by unexpected responses (such as blood pressure that drops quickly) to anaesthesia or other medications during the surgery.

- *Risk of additional surgeries*: For example, hysterectomy, bladder repair, etc.

In caesarean birth, the possible risks to the baby include the following:

- *Premature birth*: If the due date was not accurately calculated, the baby could be delivered too early.

- *Breathing problems*: Babies born by caesarean are more likely to develop breathing problems (normal labour is good for babies!)

- *Low Apgar scores*: Babies born by caesarean sometimes have low Apgar scores. The low score can be an effect of the anaesthesia and caesarean birth, or the baby may have been in distress to begin with. Or perhaps the baby was not stimulated as he or she would have been by vaginal birth.

- *Foetal injury*: Although rare, the surgeon can accidentally nick the baby while making the incision.

© *International Caesarean Awareness Network (ICAN).*
Reproduced with kind permission.

IMMEDIATE CARE AFTER A CAESAREAN

A caesarean section is a major operation, and it is going to take some time to recovery from one. You will therefore probably be kept in hospital for longer than you would if you had had a normal vaginal birth, and you will need more care from nurses and others. You will be encouraged to gently begin to get active; moving around reduces the risk of infection and prevents clots. Either later the same day or the next morning, it is a good idea to get out of bed and sit out for a time.

You will need some help in the first few days; staff are often busy, but do not be afraid to ask.

TIPS FOR RECOVERY AFTER A CAESAREAN

- *Take it slowly*. You'll probably feel like you've been hit by a bus the next day. Go easy on yourself. Just getting out of bed is going to be very painful. The midwives will want you up and about quickly; they're not doing it for kicks — it's important for you to be up and mobile to prevent blood clots. Those first few steps are going to be painful and you will need help. If you've never had surgery before, it can be a shock how your body reacts and how much it takes out of you. Take baby steps and don't rush yourself.

- *Take your pain medications.* Even if you are breastfeeding, your doctors and nurses will still urge you to take your medications. You'll feel better and you'll be more motivated to keep up the breastfeeding. The actual amount of medications that will reach your breastmilk and your baby are minimal and quite safe but be sure that your caregiver knows that you are breastfeeding. You will need those medications to help you during those first few weeks in order to walk, sleep, etc.

- *Let others help you.* Swallow your pride and let your partner, family or friends help you with the house and caring for the baby. Even a simple task like climbing into bed can make you feel 90 years old.

- *Keep your necessities close.* Having necessary items such as nappies, wipes, tissues, mobile phone, paper towels, remote control, pain medications, bottles, nipple cream, etc. close at hand will help tremendously. Having them next to you will help keep you from having to continuously get up and down or move from room to room.

- *Pulling to a sitting position.* Those tummy muscles that you once took for granted will be of no use to you for the first few weeks following your operation. To pull yourself from a lying position to a sitting one, be sure to either have someone help you or use something like the back of the couch to pull yourself up gently.

- Another good trick if you are lying on a couch or bed is to try gently rolling off it (assuming it is not too high off the ground) to the floor and then pull yourself up using a sturdy object such as a table or a nightstand.

- *Avoid stairs.* If at all possible; avoid climbing stairs for at least the first week. If your room is upstairs, set up camp downstairs on the couch.

- *Create a pillow splint.* Laughing, sneezing, coughing or taking deep breaths those first few days will be extremely painful. If you need to do any of those things, take a soft pillow and press it gently to your abdomen.

- *Avoid greasy foods and carbonated drinks*: Once your bowels begin working properly after surgery, you will be extremely gassy. Gas bubbles will wreak havoc on your sensitive insides. Be sure to avoid anything that will only irritate your bowels further.

- *Keep checking your incision*: You might not want to look at it, but keep a constant check on your incision. Your doctor will advise you on what he/she would like you to do to keep the area clean. Report any inflammation, redness or discharge.

- *Talk about your feelings*: Depending on the circumstances of your caesarean section, you will most likely have conflicting emotions surrounding the event. Top it off with the normal post-partum blues and you may feel like an emotional wreck. Talk to someone you trust about how you feel, or talk with other mothers who have experienced the same things. Don't be afraid to cry and don't feel ashamed of your feelings. It is normal to feel angry, regretful or sad about having a caesarean.

© *Jaime Warren and www.caesareanbirth.com.*
Adapted and reproduced with kind permission.

CHOOSING A CAESAREAN

More and more women are requesting caesareans in Ireland, and indeed worldwide. The reasons behind these requests include fear of vaginal birth, often after a traumatic first birth; misinformation on the risks of caesareans; and, for some, it offers a sense of control. Caesareans save lives but have become routine "procedures". The risks are well documented. It is major surgery and although it may provide a quick and relatively pain-free birth, the recovery time is often 6–8 weeks and there is an increase in complications for both mum and baby. Some choose caesareans mistakenly thinking that they are avoiding pelvic floor damage but this is often due to lifestyle and the pregnancy itself, not the birth.

A POSITIVE CAESAREAN

In the UK Professor Nick Fisk has started what he calls a "natural caesarean". This groundbreaking approach to surgical delivery — Fisk calls
it a "**skin-to-skin caesarean**" or "walking the baby out" — has been
pioneered by him partly in response to the rising caesarean rate. As
Fisk started to examine the conventions of surgical delivery, he was
struck by how easily they could be challenged. Why, for example, did
they need to be done so quickly, when slowing them down would give
the parents more chance to participate in their child's delivery and
might give the baby a gentler experience of coming into the world?
Why, too, was it so important for the parents to be screened off from
the mother's abdomen? And was it really essential for the baby to be
whisked off for an immediate medical examination, rather than delivered into the arms of his mother?

This is the birth of your child, a completely different surgical experience than any other, an experience to be treated as similarly to a
vaginal birth experience as is humanly possible.

If you do need a caesarean, then it would be better for you to receive a spinal/epidural anaesthetic and remain conscious during the operation, participating in the birth of your child.

If an emergency caesarean is necessary under general anaesthetic,
then be sure your baby is given to your partner as soon as possible after birth and held by him (hopefully next to his naked chest — skin to
skin contact) until you are awake and can be told of the baby's sex and
well-being (by your partner).

If an elective caesarean is necessary, then you should request that
you be able to begin labour naturally before the caesarean is done.
That is, you do not want a date and time preset; you wish for your
baby to decide the day on which it is ready to be born to avoid any
problems with prematurity and for both of you to reap the benefits of
your hormones.

Your baby should remain with you at all times — no disappearing off to the nursery with your partner. No matter how "nice" this is, it can affect your bonding with your new baby. If your baby must go to the nursery, then *do* send your partner and encourage the "skin-to-skin" contact mentioned before. Your baby will really be craving this contact, and he will most likely recognise your partner's voice.

Make sure theatre staff realise that you would appreciate a verbal description of the birth as it occurs. You may have previously felt left out of your past caesarean(s) as your body and labour might have been discussed as though you weren't there.

How about asking the surgeon to leave the umbilical cord long and allow the father or mother the chance to cut it? That way the parents do not miss out on the sensation or their own right to tell their story of "cutting a cord".

Would you like to meet your new baby in his/her unclothed, naked newborn state — a wet, slippery baby? Then request that the baby please be placed on your chest with a warm blanket over you both. It would do a lot to make this surgical delivery a bit more natural for mother, father and baby. And it may even resolve a few inner conflicts that are faced after the birth.

How about breastfeeding your baby straight away? Let them know that you would like to feed your baby while you are being sutured, if you feel up to it, and you would like your baby to stay with you throughout the surgery and even during the recovery. Or you could arrange for the lactation consultant of the hospital (or your own private one) to be present at the caesarean birth and bring the baby to you in recovery, to breastfeed within that first hour of birth.

Let them know that your partner would be delighted to hold his/her child within your view throughout these procedures, if you feel unable to participate in the bonding (at least you would be able to witness it this time).

You may also be able to organise with your doctor to allow a quiet relaxation CD to be played throughout the birth. Don't let it intrude on the birth, though; just enough to gently enhance the experience.

What about that placenta? Most women who birth vaginally get to see it, at least, and maybe you would like to.

Make a birth plan! Have several copies with you and give it to everyone involved in your caesarean! They won't know what is important to you unless you let them know.

Write to the Head of Obstetrics in the hospital about your birth plan. That way, they have plenty of time to fully understand what you want, as well as give them the opportunity to raise with you any concerns they may have. Once you have both reached an agreement about your caesarean then get that agreement in writing and take it with you to the hospital so staff do not have to run around and "get approval" from the appropriate person.

Ask the hospital to take you through every step of the procedure. Make sure they explain to you every light and every sound. Much of the anxiety happens when you can see flashing lights and disturbing noises and you don't know what it means.

Make sure that there is someone to take digital photos of the birth and the baby (in case you are having a general anaesthetic). Then if the baby has to be taken away for observation you can see pictures of the baby as soon as you wake from the procedure. You can use a camera phone but the quality won't be as good — but you can send it to friends and family immediately.

After being wheeled into the recovery room, ask that they dim the lights for you and your baby. (This might not be possible, especially if you have a few other patients in the recovery ward and checks requiring observations are being done all the time).

You might want a special blanket to wrap baby in while waiting with you at recovery. Note that if your baby is with you at recovery, most hospitals will require a midwife to be in attendance. This is why it's a good idea to get the head of maternity and operating theatre involved very early, to assist with staffing requirements.

VBAC: VAGINAL BIRTH AFTER CAESAREAN

The old adage "once a caesarean always a caesarean" is no longer holding true for more and more women giving birth. Worldwide VBAC (vaginal birth after caesarean) births are increasing. As women become better educated in the birthing process, more are opting for labour instead of automatically scheduling a repeat caesarean.

Is VBAC Safe?

It is possible for most women who have had a caesarean (70 to 80 per cent) to go on to have a successful vaginal birth. There is a very small risk (5 per 1,000) of uterine rupture with one low transverse scar. (most caesarean sections are performed using a cut below the bikini line; it is less disfiguring and takes less time to recover from than the previous cut from a mother's navel to her pubic bone).

Why Choose VBAC?

According to Birthrites.org, "There are many psychological effects of a caesarean birth. These continue on if the caesarean was unexpected by the mother. The loss of control, and the fear associated with an earlier birth experience, may result in the need to maintain control the next time. The amount of technology involved and the sterile atmosphere may cause a desire for a 'natural' labour and a reduction in unnecessary interventions. When women choose a VBAC birth, they tend to be making a highly informed choice."

QUESTIONS ABOUT VBAC

Q: My doctor told me my pelvis is too small to vaginally deliver a baby over eight pounds and I have to have another caesarean. Is this true?

A: No, the pelvis and the baby's head are not fixed bone structures. During labour the pelvis opens, allowing room for the baby, whose head moulds to fit. Your baby's head is made up of five quite pliable bone "plates" that overlap each other while moving through the birth canal. You've probably seen pictures of babies with cone-shaped heads. This isn't permanent; the bones will return to their prebirth state within a few hours.

The pelvis will actually open up 33 per cent larger than its pre-pregnant size with a squatting position. There are several factors that contribute to this. First a hormone called relaxin is released during the latter part of pregnancy, which softens the ligaments and cartilage surrounding the pelvis.

You may notice this during pregnancy; it can feel like arthritis in your joints. Also, different positions assumed during labour, such as walking, climbing stairs and squatting, will change the dimensions of the pelvis. This combined with the flexibility of the baby's head gives ample room for babies to move through the pelvis.

Q: I can't find a doctor willing to support a vaginal birth after caesarean.

A: Finding a doctor to be supportive can be difficult. Take the time to make an appointment and go and see several doctors. Ask questions and listen to their answers. VBACs can take a lot of work — even before labour.

Q: Doesn't a vaginal birth cause problems like pelvic floor "damage"?

A: Lead researcher Dr Alastair MacLennan in an interview with Reuters Health states: "80% of the problems a woman having a vaginal delivery has, also happen to a woman having a caesarean section." Most often it is the interventions like episiotomies, vacuum and forceps deliveries that contribute to urinary and faecal incontinence, uterine prolapse, and pelvic floor damage, rather than the vaginal birth itself. Women who have had caesarean deliveries also experience urinary and faecal incontinence and other concerns due to the surgery or simply as a result of the hormones of pregnancy and/or the drugs used during the delivery.

Q: Wouldn't a caesarean be safer than a vaginal birth after a caesarean?

A: A caesarean section is major abdominal surgery, with all that entails. The surgery itself, as opposed to medical problems that might lead to a caesarean, increases the risk of maternal death, hysterectomy, haemorrhage, infection, blood clots, damage to blood vessels, urinary bladder and other organs, postpartum depression, post-traumatic stress syndrome, and re-hospitalisation for complications.

Potential chronic complications from scar tissue adhesions include pelvic pain, bowel problems, and pain during sexual intercourse. Scar tissue makes subsequent caesareans more difficult to perform, increasing the risk of injury to other organs as well as placenta previa, placenta accreta, infertility, ectopic pregnancy, uterine rupture in subsequent pregnancies and the risk of chronic problems from adhesions.

There are also risks to the baby such as respiratory distress syndrome, prematurity, lower birth weights, jaundice and lower Apgar scores.

© International Caesarean Awareness Network (ICAN).
Reproduced with kind permission.

Since we know that vaginal deliveries are almost always safer for the mother, and usually as safe for the baby, and that VBAC attempts are successful in about 80 per cent of cases, why do some women still choose to have a repeat caesarean rather than try for a vaginal delivery? In some cases it is fear of pain during labour (although many patients report that the pain from recuperation from a caesarean section is worse than labour pain); in others it is a "fear of the unknown"; while for some women there is a convenience in scheduling the exact date of their baby's birth. Often a mother who has had a traumatic induction that ended in a caesarean will probably *not* want to repeat that experience and not even consider VBAC — without even realising that the induction itself may well have led to the caesarean.

Finally, a number of women do not wish to take the risk, no matter how rare, of uterine rupture. No matter what the reason, since there is a small risk with an attempt at vaginal delivery and a risk with repeat caesarean, women should make the best choice for themselves, based on their specific medical history and individual situation.

I run the Irish ICAN (International Caesarean Awareness Network) chapter, a support group for women who have been negatively affected by caesareans. Come along to a meeting and find out how you can help yourself and others who've been through the same experience.

VBAC Birth Plan

Labour:

- I would prefer not to have routine vaginal exams except on admission.

- I would appreciate unrestricted movement and positions throughout my labour.

- No arbitrary time limits to give birth as long as my baby and I are doing well.

- I would like to avoid any artificial speeding up of my labour.

- Please leave my membranes intact to rupture spontaneously.

- Pain relief by relaxation, shower, walking and other movement and position changes, adequate nutrition by mouth. If I change my mind about pain relief, I will let my midwife know.

Birth:

- I prefer to choose my own position for birth.

- Please do not rush the pushing stage; I would like to birth at my own pace with no time limits as long as baby and I are doing well.

- Allow my baby to clear own mucous naturally rather than with routine suctioning.

- I would like skin-to-skin contact with my baby immediately following birth.

- Please allow the cord to stop pulsating completely before any clamping, cutting or administration of medications to me.

- Please allow for breastfeeding and natural separation of placenta; no speeding up of placenta delivery.

- I would prefer no manual exploration of uterus after birth.

We recognise that true emergencies do sometimes arise and will be relying upon your skill in the event of such a circumstance. We hope to have full communication in that case, with you informing us of all our options.

The Times They Are a-Changin':
New Developments in
Maternity Care

Domino Scheme

Some hospitals in Ireland now offer more flexibility in their maternity services, operating early discharge schemes, home births (also known as "*domino deliveries*") and midwives' clinics. These are largely pilot schemes at present. (Personally I believe pizzas and packages are delivered; babies are *birthed*.) You have to fulfil certain criteria to be eligible for some of the schemes.

Several maternity hospitals are currently operating a **Domino/** Home Birth Scheme in certain parts of the country. This scheme enables a few women who are deemed at "low risk of complications" to see members of a dedicated midwives' team for their antenatal visits and to have a member of this team deliver their baby, either at home or in hospital. Antenatal visits are made either to the Community Midwives' Clinic or to certain local health centres and with your GP if you are doing combined care. Additional visits are made to the woman's home. Each woman interested in the Domino/Home Birth Scheme will have a routine scan at around 18–22 weeks and a physical examination and history-taking to make sure you're suitable for the scheme. If any problems develop during the pregnancy or in labour, you will be immediately transferred back to full hosptial care (around 31 per cent of cases are transferred — the criteria for transfer are very strict). Under the Domino/Home Birth Scheme, you are entitled to an early discharge after birth, if you wish, and the midwife will visit you at home for up to a week after the birth. The scheme is free.

EARLY TRANSFER HOME SCHEME

This service gives new mothers the opportunity to go home within the first 36 hours following delivery — as early as six hours after the birth in some hospitals. This can be great for some women but for many first-time mums it can be terrifying. It's limited to certain areas so check with your hospital to see what is available in your area. You will be visited on a daily basis by a community midwife until your baby is five days old.

You will be released from hospital six hours following your baby's birth. The Early Transfer Home Community Midwives provide care during the antenatal period and in the days following delivery. You can opt for combined antenatal care between your obstetrician and community midwife if that suits you better.

After you have given birth you will be transferred to the postnatal ward to rest and enjoy your new addition. Let your midwives know if you would like to be discharged early. Women who go home on their first day following delivery will receive approximately four visits, while those who go home on day two will receive approximately three visits. Generally, you will be visited by the same midwife postnatally. The midwives will check both you and your baby to ensure you are both well. They offer feeding advice and support, monitor baby's weight and do the heel prick test.

Another guide to maternity services in Ireland is produced by Cuidiu: The Irish Childbirth Trust. It is entitled *Consumer Guide to Maternity Services in Ireland*, and is available from Cuidiu. Cuidiu is a parent-to-parent community-based voluntary support group.

These schemes are available free of charge.

MIDWIFE-LED SERVICES

Midwife-led care is the ideal model of care for most women having a normal pregnancy. Women who attend midwives throughout their pregnancies tend to have fewer interventions and have a lower chance of ending up with a caesarean. You'll get to know a small group of midwives throughout your pregnancy, so you'll already know the midwife who takes care of you when you have your baby. **Midwife led units (MLUs)** are supportive of active birth and have birthing pools. The rooms are set up more like a comfy hotel room than a sterile hospital, with any equipment discreetly hidden away in wardrobes. You'll be encouraged to use birth mats, exercise birth balls and, importantly, you are free to labour and birth in whatever position you want. In the unlikely event of there being a complication, there is always a consultant and paediatric team on call. You are free to go home as early as six hours after the birth and have home visits from the midwives. There are currently only two MLUs in Ireland, one in Cavan and another in Drogheda, both pilot programmes. Check the small print for guidelines — it can be like trying to get a Willy Wonka ticket to get a spot on these pilot programmes!

DOULAS DO WHAT?

A relatively new trend in Irish maternity care is the arrival of the birth **doula** or professional labour supporter. The doula's primary objective is to nurture and protect the mother's memory of her birth experience through education, physical and emotional support. The doula does not try to enforce birth plans or "advocate" for the parents — that has to come from the parents themselves — but they help parents ask the right questions. The doula empowers the parents with the knowledge to make choices that are important to them and the confidence to communicate effectively with their caregiver and the hospital staff. Doulas work with the hospital staff and can free up midwives to attend to women who need more care. While consultants, midwives and nurses have other labouring women to look after, doula support is constant throughout labour and birth, beginning in the home.

In 1989, the research team of Klaus, Kennell and Klaus did a large-scale study to investigate the use of continuous one-on-one support in labour. From the study of over 600 normal labours, they found that the use of a doula made a tremendous difference in the outcome of the birth experience. The benefits of doula support as reported by Klaus et al. included:

- 25 per cent shorter labours (by two hours minimum);

- 50 per cent fewer caesarean sections;

- 40 per cent fewer epidurals

- 30 to 40 per cent decrease in the need for forceps, vacuum extraction, pitocin and narcotics.

Statistics also show that women who have positive memories of their birth are less likely to develop post-partum depression, are more positive about their babies, and are more confident in their ability to be good mothers. What a great start to your transition to motherhood!

GIVING BIRTH AT HOME

Home births are on the rise, but arranging a home birth in Ireland isn't easy. We have a severe shortage of community/independent midwives and there are very few GPs who will attend a home birth. Check with your local HSE Area (formerly Health Boards) to find out what's available in your area. Where a woman chooses to have a home birth and the HSE Area cannot provide the service, some HSE Areas provide a home birth grant towards the cost of contracting the services of a private midwife. These days you almost need to hire your midwife *before* you get pregnant!

Write to your local HSE Area's Community Care Section informing them of your wish for a home birth, and requesting a list of midwives in your area. Or contact the Home Birth Association who will have all the latest and best information. Unfortunately, home birth is still not the norm in Ireland so your HSE Area may not even be as clued in as the HBA.

When you make contact with the midwife or doctor of your choice, you will need to ask them to fill out a *Form of Application for Maternity Care*. This will entitle you to free antenatal, delivery and postnatal services. The HSE Area will also provide you with a "maternity pack", with all you should need for a home birth.

Alternatively, you can hire a midwife privately and your antenatal, delivery and postnatal care will be provided by her. Where a woman engages the services of a private midwife for the purpose of a home birth, her HSE Area may make a contribution towards the costs incurred. For a list of independent midwives, contact the Homebirth Association of Ireland. (See also the Domino scheme, as discussed on page 141.)

THE MODERN McBIRTH

by Sheila Stubbs

Hospitals are often said to be good places to give birth because of their facilities. They are well equipped and have everything a birthing couple might need readily available. But so what?

In the restaurant business, particularly the fast-food business, kitchens are designed specifically for efficient food production in order to serve the most customers with the least effort in the least amount of time. But this doesn't mean we need the same equipment to prepare meals at home! Admittedly, many of us enjoy the familiar and when we go to these restaurants we know ahead of time exactly what we will get. We also know what we will get in the hospital, since it's pretty much standard fare in all franchises. There is some variety to the menu, but you're in trouble if you find yourself in a burger place when you have your heart set on a stir-fry. Birth shouldn't have to be like a drive-thru window. "Let's see, you ordered the birthing room with a jacuzzi, and you'll need an epidural to go. You want pitocin with that?"

When you go in for your McBirth at the local franchise, you know what to expect. Nurses and doctors are there to serve you, but special orders may upset them. After all, this is *their* territory, and *they* are in charge. Because you are in their territory, you have few rights and little to do but pace the halls or lie on the assigned bed. You might be allowed to shower, but any staff member is free to walk in on you at any time.

By contrast, home birth can be like a take-out Chinese. You can sit around in your underwear or stark naked, lie down, sit, squat, dance, watch TV. Some couples prefer the quiet candlelight-and-wine atmosphere, listening to soft music while they wait until the bun is ready to come out of the oven.

Other home-birthing couples have a Birth Day Party. Just like any family celebration, there are balloons, gift-wrapped surprises for everyone, cake and champagne! The cake is prepared ahead of time, decorated and put in the freezer. The presents are bought and wrapped and waiting for the Birth Day before they can be opened, the same as we anticipate Christmas Day.

Many women find they enjoy getting ready for the baby and the celebration party afterwards to help pass the time during labour. The nice thing is, it all depends on what *you* want. You can call someone over to be with you to help out, or be alone; it's up to you. It's your house, and you don't have to ask permission or argue policy with anyone!

Depending on how you feel, you can spend the hours of your labour making sure the laundry is all caught up, the house is tidy, and the next meal is planned. If you don't feel up to it, of course, you don't have to do anything. But it is somehow emotionally satisfying to complete these "nesting behaviours" yourself, such as putting clean sheets on the bed, setting out the new baby's clothes, and boiling scissors to sterilize them for cutting the cord. It's exciting to get the baby's tiny clothes and nappies laid out, reminding you with each contraction that you will soon have a real, live baby wearing them!

When you birth at home, you don't have the concern about when to go to the hospital hanging over your head. Go too soon, and you'll have a long time to labour in a crowded ward, waiting for full dilation, waiting for permission to push. And without a doubt, the longer you are there, the more likely you are to have some interventions to "speed things up". Go too late and you'll have to deal with those horrendous contractions in the car; every little bump in the road is magnified so that a smooth ride seems like torture. Then you'll be asked to cooperate with admission procedures, signing papers, undressing, being examined and settled into a room when your contractions are demanding all your attention.

Believe it or not, the reason women have less need for pain relief at home birth is because of the ideas mentioned above. The midwives are the ones in an unfamiliar territory! In her own home the woman feels in control of her environment and her situation. Giving birth is perceived to be something she "does", not something that happens to her. That perception of personal power can be enough to help her handle the amazing power of contractions. Drugs? Who needs them!

Your house may not have the same set-up as the McBirth franchise, but it doesn't matter. The homemade quality and ambiance are unsurpassed.

HOME BIRTH CARE

Ask any mother who has had a home birth and the first thing they'll tell you is how great it is to *not* have to sit around hospitals for hours waiting on appointments and how they were able to get into their own bed (use their own shower) right after their baby was born. You don't have to go anywhere for antenatal visits; the midwife will come to your home — shocking, eh? Visits will last about an hour and are very easy going with lots of opportunity to get to know each other over a cup of tea, discuss birth plans and ask questions. You will get to know your midwife (midwives if in a joint/group practice) very well, and you will have the comfort of knowing she will be the one with you at the birth.

Some home birth midwives aren't comfortable with mothers giving birth in a pool. If that's important to you, then have a chat with another midwife (but be aware your choices are limited). Your partner and other children can be present and involved in the new baby's progress.

There are fewer routine high technology antenatal screenings (ultrasound scans, etc.). These can of course be arranged through a hospital if required. Your midwife is a trusted health professional available to you by telephone at all times.

Benefits of Home Birth Aftercare

- You or your partner and other family members will be able to stay together with your baby — in bed with a cup of tea and a packet of Hobnobs.

- Your other children won't be wondering where mum has disappeared to (gone to hospital).

- No routine procedures or arguing hospital policies — you're the boss!

- All postnatal visits (baby checks and six-week checks of mother and infant) are in the privacy of your own home.

Home Birth Midwives and Hospital Midwives: What's the Difference?

Midwifery is a profession, totally independent of nursing (although in Ireland it used to be the case that anybody who wanted to become a midwife would have to complete training as a nurse first). Practising independent midwives are able to take sole responsibility for the care of mainly healthy women and babies, whereas nurses care for sick people, usually under the direction of doctors. (Remember, you are pregnant, not ill.) Your midwife is the specialist in *normal* maternity care. I know I keep repeating this, but it's important: most women (80 per cent or more) have problem-free pregnancies and labours. Your midwife is trained to be able to recognise possible problems early on. If a problem does come up, your midwife will arrange a transfer to the hospital. Hospital midwives don't get to see a lot of normal births; they do see lots of inductions, epidurals and episiotomies — so no wonder some of them see birth as a medical condition. If that was all you are exposed to, then that's your reality.

Is Home Birth Safe?

Yes. Home birth is a prime example of how our actions are affected (or not) by factual realities (scientific data) or perceptual reality (beliefs). When someone mentions home birth, do you automatically think to yourself *"How irresponsible — what if something goes wrong?"* or do you think *"Excellent; this woman knows her stuff"*? For the majority it's probably the former. Many people ask if home birth is safe. Our society views labour and birth as an illness or medical condition that needs to be fixed or cured. Since the beginning of time, we have given birth without medical help or intervention.

The World Health Organisation (WHO) says:

> It has never been scientifically proven that the hospital is a safer place than home for a woman who has had an uncomplicated pregnancy to have her baby. Studies of planned home births in developed countries with women who have had uncomplicated pregnancies have shown sickness and death rates for mother and baby *equal to or better* than hospital birth statistics for women with uncomplicated pregnancies.

So are you perfectly safe delivering at home? Carl Jones (author of *Childbirth Choices Today*) states:

> There is always going to be some risk when giving birth, as in all of life, and women should be carefully screened for any health problems that could be dangerous during labour and delivery. For certain women in rare circumstances, obstetric care is essential. However, for most women, better, healthier results are seen when mothers choose to birth at home.

If you are a woman with no health problems or contraindications to safe labour and delivery, consider birthing at home. The risks to you and your baby are lower at home.

NEED AN EXTRA $25,000?

Jock Doubleday, a birth activist from the US, made this offer recently:

I Jock Doubleday, will pay $25,000.00 (US) to the first person who sends me, both by email and postal mail, a study published in an industry journal in any country, in any time period, demonstrating hospital birth to be safer, in any category (i.e., infant or maternal mortality or morbidity), for most mothers and babies than home birth with a trained midwife in attendance. The term "midwife" does not include Certified Nurse Midwives, who, because of their conventional medical training, and in spite of their good intentions, may bring the fear-based medical model of childbirth with them into the home, thus skewing home birth data toward the technological. Fear, in any guise, is contagious. This offer has no expiration date and supersedes all previous offers of a similar nature. Contact: jockdoubleday@aol.com

---

So why is there still an assumption that hospital is safer than home? The fact is, supporters of active management of labour point to the fact that, in the past, where fewer interventions were available, mortality rates for mothers and newborns were much higher. But this is really accounted for by improvements in living standards, nutrition, general health and antenatal care; and these factors apply equally as well to hospital as home births.

In the UK the perinatal mortality rate for home birth compares very favourably with that of births in general:

- *Home births*: 4-5 in 1000

- *Hospital births*: 9-10 in 1000.

The following quote is from the *UK Health Committee Second Report House of Commons: Maternity Services, Vol. 1 (The Winterton Report)*, published in March 1992:

> On the basis of what we have heard, the committee must draw the conclusion that the policy of encouraging all women to give birth in hospital cannot be justified on grounds of safety.

The *British Medical Journal* of 23 November 1996 published a Swiss study "Home vs. Hospital deliveries: follow up study of matched pairs for procedures and outcome". Their key conclusions include:

> There are no obvious disadvantages of home delivery for mother or child when the mother opts for home delivery.

A landmark study released in 2005 again backed up all the positive recommendations about home birth and safety ("Outcomes of planned home births with certified professional midwives: large prospective study in North America", Kenneth C. Johnson, senior epidemiologist, Betty-Anne Daviss, project manager, *BMJ*, 2005, 330:1416 (18 June), doi:10.1136/bmj.330.7505.1416.

In some areas of Ireland, mothers-to-be have to make round trips of 100 miles to attend antenatal clinics in hospital. This is due to closures of smaller maternity units and the running down of domiciliary services.

Apart from the obvious inconvenience of travelling such distances, there are other risks involved — long and high-speed car journeys to hospital; giving birth unattended either at home or on the roadside, which is particularly applicable on second or subsequent babies, where labours can be very short and fast.

Given these risks, some women choose induction in order to avoid either of these scenarios. Inductions themselves come with risks, so it becomes a Catch-22 situation: take the "risk" of having a home birth, which has been proven safe for most women; or make your life miserable by racing to a hospital mid-labour; or opt for an unnecessary early induction that might not work! In these cases, it makes sense to have your baby at home with a local midwife (provided you can find one).

Benefits of Having a Home Birth:

- You're in your own home; it doesn't get any better than that!

- If you have other children they can be at the birth, as can your partner, sister, best friend or even great-granny!

- Nobody will be watching the clock or trying to rush your labour.

- You have your baby your way; no wondering if you are "allowed" to birth on the floor or swinging from the chandeliers if that's what floats your boat.

- You can labour in a birth pool.

- No routine procedures.

- You'll be more relaxed (less adrenaline) so your body will labour more effectively.

All of these benefits also reduce complications in childbirth for you and your baby: less foetal distress diagnoses; fewer babies needing resuscitation; fewer low Apgar scores at one minute (a check on the baby's well-being); less incidence of post-partum haemorrhage in the mother.

MARIA'S BIRTH STORY

I was eight days overdue for the birth of my second child. We had planned a home birth in my mom's house, as this put us in the catchment area for the Community Midwives from the National Maternity Hospital. This was to be my partner's first birth experience and our six-year-old daughter was very excited and prepared.

I had spent the last two days with mild contractions during the day, getting stronger towards the evening, but then stopping throughout the night — quite frustrating. I had been leaking a bit of amniotic fluid, but the midwives had said the forewaters were intact and that perhaps it was a small leak from the hindwaters but that I could still wait until things kick-started. I had recently been stuck in traffic for two hours, so we decided to stay over in mom's, just in case.

On the Friday I woke up at 5.30 am, having had the best night's sleep in ages. I left Paul and Ella to sleep. Contractions started coming every five to six minutes, about 45 seconds long and more significant than the ones the previous days, so I rocked on the birth ball in the living room.

At about 6.00 am Paul woke up and joined me, He rubbed my back as I rocked. My mom woke up at about 7.00, and moved a still sleeping Ellie from the bed we were planning to use, which was a double-bed mattress on the floor in the dining room. Paul called the midwives who said that the new shift midwife would be there shortly and that she would call back when she arrived.

She did call at 7.30 and said that she and her second midwife were going to leave for us straight away. I was in the bath while Paul talked to them, and mom poured water across my tummy. The contractions were coming hot and heavy and I started to find the bath too restrictive and was unable to kneel on all fours, my more comfortable position. I went back downstairs and knelt on the mattress on the floor, leaning over the birth ball. Ella had woken by now and came in to give me a kiss. She asked if I was OK and I said, yes, baby will be here soon, and she said that she and Grandma were going to go make the baby a birthday cake and card.

At 8.15 the midwife called again, asking if everything was OK, and letting us know she was ten minutes away. Paul was rubbing my back and reassuring me, "They'll be here soon." — between bouts of muttering, "Where the *#$* are they?"

At about 8.30 the contractions changed, I felt the overwhelming urge to push, I pushed away the birth ball. I needed solid ground. "Stop," I told Paul who was rubbing my back. I felt I needed to make sure that it was time to push without any other stimulus. "That was different; I have to push."

I had been hoping that the midwives would get there in time but now I knew that we were on our own. I felt a panic, for Paul; how would he cope with this? Then I had to settle down to do the job. My waters broke, I heard Paul call my mom for towels. As mom walked into the room with the towels, I heard Paul exclaim, "I can see the head!" It seemed like only a couple more pushes until Paul said, "The head's out, what do I do?"

"Is there a cord?" I asked. He said he could see one. Two more pushes and out came baby, caught by Paul's able hands.

I was still on all fours. Paul told me to lie down but I couldn't, I was too wobbly. He had to tip me over onto my side, then he handed me the baby and threw a blanket over us, and lay down beside me. We lay there quietly looking at the baby, who had opened its eyes and whimpered a bit.

Mom and Ella came in. Ella cleaned a small patch on the baby's head and kissed it, then lay down beside us. We then realised that we didn't know what sex the baby was. It was a girl; I had been sure that it was going to be a boy but Paul and Ella had chosen a girl's name, Abby Anna.

The midwife arrived ten minutes later, 9.00. My mom met them at the door saying, "She's here," to which the midwife replied, "Oh yes, I'm sorry were late." Mom said, "No, the baby — she's here!"

The midwives came in and sat watching us for another ten minutes before they did anything, just chatting, helping to get baby latched on, and looking, taking in the information. I was happy they didn't come in and "take over". They then cut the cord, but I would have wanted them to offer it to Paul to do, a last final job to do. Then they checked and weighed Abby, 8 lbs 11 oz, and helped Patrick to dress her and also helped me to birth the placenta and checked the perineum for any damage, helped me clean up, have a shower, etc.

I spent the rest of that day in bed. I felt great and my family kept saying how great I looked. It was so nice to have Ella there too. Next time she wants to be in the room for the birth. Paul, at this time, had lost his knees, he kept saying, "But what if something had gone wrong?" It took him a long time to get over that shock. Even now, he doesn't like to think about what might have been. He has agreed to go for a home birth again next time — but this time with the midwife!

I felt and still feel completely empowered by this experience; this is what my body is made to do and I did it without any medical involvement. I often wonder how many other births become medicalised when, if left to instinct they would have turned out as well as my experience. I'm dying to do it all again; I'm afraid I could get addicted to being pregnant, giving birth and having children!

LOTUS BIRTH

By Sarah Buckley

Lotus birth is the practice of leaving the umbilical cord uncut, so that the baby remains attached to his/her placenta until the cord naturally separates at the umbilicus — exactly as a cut cord does — at three to ten days after birth. This prolonged contact can be seen as a time of transition, allowing the baby to slowly and gently let go of his/her attachment to the mother's body.

Although we have no written records of cultures that leave the cord uncut, many cultures hold the placenta in high esteem. For example, Maori people from New Zealand bury the placenta ritually on the ancestral *marae*, and the Hmong, a hill tribe from South East Asia, believe that the placenta must be retrieved after death to ensure physical integrity in the next life: a Hmong baby's placenta is buried inside the house of its birth.

Things to consider if you're planning a Lotus birth.

- *"Uggggggh . . ."* is a typical response, and you'll get sick of hearing it very quickly! It might be easier to not tell anyone. Many couples who plan lotus birth see the days with the placenta (usually four to six days) as private family time and make a rule that they will not have guests until the placenta is separated. This relieves the new mother of performance anxiety as she gets to know her new baby. It gives the baby a quiet transition period to intensively bond with his/her parents. One couple I know did not let anyone know their baby had been born until the placenta had separated naturally.

- *What if it smells terrible?* Ground rosemary sprinkled all over the surfaces gives the placenta a pleasant smell like turkey stuffing. (Hope you're feeling festive!) There *will* be a smell. It is not terrible. A cake rack can be helpful to place the placenta on to allow air to circulate. Nappies are helpful to prevent bedclothes from being stained with blood. The placenta is organ meat that is fresher than any meat you have ever purchased. It will naturally begin to smell after a few days of being in the air. Sometimes keeping it in a casserole dish in cold water can help too.

- *What if I decide not to do it once I've started?* Not a problem. The cord can be cut at any time and usually is atrophied (dried and shrunk) enough that it needs no clamp after 24 hours. It is common for new parents to go through periods where they think Lotus birth is just too much trouble. Often the mother wants to give up and cut the cord and the father will talk her into persisting a while longer; then, the father can be fed up and the mother will encourage him to keep going. It becomes a quiet meditation to wait vigilantly for the cord to fall and in our fast-moving society it is a real contest to slow down for the baby. Parents report that the days spent with the placenta attached taught them a great deal about cooperative parenting and patience.

- *What are the annoying aspects of Lotus birth?* It can seem like a nuisance to have to move the placenta every time you move the baby. Having a piece of raw meat in your family bed is a little peculiar, too, and can be messy. Once the cord dries after 24 hours, it has the consistency of rawhide, which makes it seem like your baby has a wire coat hanger protruding from his/her belly. None of these problems is insurmountable if the parents can be relaxed, stay close to bed and view Lotus Birth as a rite of passage.

- *How do I do this with a three-year-old jumping around on the bed?* This is actually one of the biggest challenges and is a reason that Lotus birth most often happens with first births. Protecting the newborn from the exuberance of a three-year-old is not easy at the best of times. Prior to the birth, the parents should put some thought into creating a "nest" for the new baby and mom for the Lotus time. The father and older child can build a "play space" of some kind with new library books and music for nap times. Enlisting friends and family to take the older child for some active outdoor fun each day will also help the new parents maintain the sanctity of the Lotus time for the baby.

© *Reproduced with kind permission of Sarah Buckley and Birthlove.com*

WATER BIRTH

In the same way that a nice soak in a warm bath can melt away muscle tension and the stress of the day, using warm water in labour has a wonderful effect and allows for a more gentle entry into the world for your baby. Michel Odent pioneered the birth pool in France in the early 1960s and the use of birthing pools has grown steadily ever since. Using water during labour helps relax you so labour can progress normally. It takes the weight off your limbs so you can change positions very easily and the water makes you feel much lighter (can't be a bad thing when you've been pregnant for nine or even ten months). If you're planning a home birth then getting a pool these days is very easy. Birth pools come in all shapes and sizes — the deeper the better.

Take a wander through your house to decide where to put your birth pool. Most mums like to labour in an enclosed area that is not too big — so right in the middle of the living room might not feel like the best place during labour. If you're birthing upstairs, then make sure your floor can take the weight of the water! You will probably also want to avoid any rooms with brand new white or light-coloured carpet. The room should be big enough so that your midwife can have easy access if needs be.

Depending on your heating system, you may need to keep the immersion on permanently so you can be sure the pool is warm enough. Ideally, the water should be maintained around 37 degrees Celsius and no higher; otherwise you're likely to get dizzy and it can affect the baby.

If you don't have a birth pool, your bathtub will do but it's not ideal. You'll want to be sure that you have someone with you to help you in and out, and a non-slip mat. The tub is a bit of a tight squeeze if your partner or other children wanted to join you.

In Russia you can even hire transparent acrylic pools. The video *Birth into Being* follows several midwives who host a "birth camp" at the edge of the Black Sea each summer; the babies are born into the warm ocean. I can't see many Irish mothers blazing a trail to Dollymount to give birth!

The recommended rental period is for four weeks — two weeks before and after estimated date of arrival. The cost is approximately €120. If using a pool with a disposable liner, you buy this for around €40. It is now also possible to purchase one-time use pools for €57. Delivery can be arranged for about €43. Check on e-Bay too; you might get a bargain.

Talk to your midwife about your plans to use a birth pool. Find out if she has had previous experience and how she feels about birthing in the water as opposed to only labouring in water (if this is your choice). If you are planning to use a pool don't focus completely on giving birth in the water. Some mothers like to get out of the water and birth "on dry land'. You won't know how you will feel until you get to that stage but don't make it a project *just* so you can have a water birth. As with the rest of labour, if it feels right then listen to what your body is telling you.

TIPS FOR GETTING READY

Put a plastic tarp under the pool. You can also use a flannel-backed vinyl tablecloth (flannel side up) under the pool, especially the side you will be getting in/out of most, to stop you slipping. Throw down a few sheets or towels on top of the tarp. Give your local St Vincent de Paul a call and get some old sheets/towels from them. You'll just be throwing them out anyway, so you won't want to use your good linen!

When using an inflatable pool, *put the cold water in first — then the hot water*. Get a thermometer (buy one that you can use for your newborn's bathtime) to test the temperature. Always fill it a quarter of the way with room temperature water, *then* add your hot water. You need to keep the temperature around 37 degrees celsius. This will keep the plastic in the tub from melting (a high priority!) and enable you to monitor the temperature of the water better. Keep an eye on the temperature coming out of the hose, too, to make sure your water heater isn't out of hot water!

It's vital to stay well hydrated and get out of the pool if you get dizzy or lightheaded. Keep a few ice cold washcloths by the pool and in the fridge. Have a few fruit juice and water ice pops already made in the freezer (you probably won't be in the mood for a Wibbly Wobbly Wonder). Keep a bowl of ice with just a bit of water that you can put a couple of washcloths in — your body temperature will warm up those cloths quickly, so get your partner to change them often!

It's better to avoid putting any aromatherapy oils in the pool. An option is to have a mister (spray bottle) with some cool, distilled water and a few drops of essential oil instead. It's much easier to get rid of a spray bottle than to have the entire house smelling of lavender from the steam of the tub and in the birth tub itself. And it can make you sick, as your sense of smell is heightened during labour.

© Pamela Hines-Powell and Circle of Life Midwifery,
www.midwifemama.com. Reproduced with kind permission.

What is the Baby's Experience of Being Born in Water?

Being born in water makes birth a very gentle process for your baby. He will not take his first breath until he reaches the surface, so there's no need to worry about your baby drowning. As far as he's concerned, he's still just floating in amniotic fluid — except that the womb just got a whole lot bigger! Birthing in the pool makes it easier to catch your own baby too (often with the guidance of your midwife). Research has shown that being born in water is a safe alternative for low-risk mothers with no medical issues (as long as mum and baby are doing well).

THE THIRD STAGE OF LABOUR

The first few hours after birth is a critical time for you and your baby to get to know each other. Coincidentally, it's within the first hour of birth that your baby is most alert and this is the best time to start breastfeeding. What you and your baby need most from each other at this time is eye contact, skin-to-skin contact and lots of cuddles. This is a brand new world to your baby so he has a lot to get used to very quickly but you can make the transition easier by keeping your baby with you. Many hospitals now see the benefits of "rooming-in" instead of automatically sending your baby to the nursery unless there is a medical need. If your baby has to go to the nursery, have your partner go with him. Co-sleeping is not encouraged in hospitals especially if the mum has had a tiring labour and is taking medication. Co-sleeping is fantastic for breastfeeding once you get home, as it means you'll get more sleep and feel better rested during the day. It's sometimes referred to as "dreamfeeding".

THE THIRD STAGE: DELIVERING THE PLACENTA

The **third stage of labour** refers to the part of labour and delivery most people forget — the birth of the placenta. As with most areas of labour, you have the choice of delivering the placenta naturally or having an actively managed third stage.

An actively managed third stage involves an injection of syntometrine into the mother's thigh. A risk of a managed third stage is that it can sometimes cause the uterus to clamp shut before the placenta has been born.

A natural third stage occurs when no drugs are administered and the baby's suckling results in the release of oxytocin, which causes the uterus to contract. As long as the placenta separates from the uterine wall, there is no rush to deliver it, as once it has peeled away from the wall of the uterus, there is no danger of haemorrhage. A doctor or midwife can easily tell whether or not the placenta has separated by gently palpating the fundus (top of the uterus). If the cord does not move, then the placenta has indeed separated from the uterine wall.

There is no need to cut the cord until the placenta has been delivered, unless it is not long enough to allow the baby to suckle, or it has become wrapped around the baby's neck in several loops. In the latter case, most of the time the cord can just be unlooped (it's quite common for a baby to be born with the cord around his neck and is easily fixed)

In most instances, the placenta will be delivered within an hour after birth. At a birth I recently supported, the placenta did not birth until 28 hours later! The mother had a great hands-off consultant who was happy to leave things alone as long as there were no signs of infection or excess bleeding. I had read about rare cases of the placenta not birthing for 12 hours, but I think this was a new record.

CARE OF THE CORD

The umbilical cord carries blood from the placenta to the newborn, and continues to do so until the cord has stopped pulsating. It is therefore not a good idea to cut the cord before it has stopped pulsating. The cord will usually stop pulsating in about 5 minutes. Policy in most Irish hospitals is to cut the cord immediately.

Once the cord has been successfully cut and clamped, there is no need to give it any special care. Cord spirit, for example, is entirely unnecessary and can even irritate the baby's skin. If anything, just apply a few drops of breastmilk to the site — this will stave off infection and will be kind to your baby's skin.

CORD STEM CELL COLLECTION

Another new option in Ireland for parents is cord stem cell collection. If you decide to preserve your baby's stem cells then you need to also look at the risks to him of early cord cutting which reduces your baby's blood volume significantly.

STEM CELLS: WHAT ARE THEY USED FOR?

Stem cells have proven their use in treating a growing number of serious, life-threatening diseases. Until recently, in the case of malignant blood disorders such as leukaemia, doctors could only hope for a bone marrow transplant in order to boost the number of healthy blood cells in the patient. However, bone marrow transplants are not always possible. The injection of stem cells has been shown to be a valid alternative to bone marrow transplants, especially in children and adolescents.

The advantage of preserving cord blood stem cells is: (a) their immediate availability, even years later; (b) there is no risk of rejection, as the healing cells are one's own; and (c) the whole process is entirely safe and drug- free. As such, it builds on a natural process.

At the moment it is believed that stem cells will play a major role in various medical fields. Stem cells lead to the renewal of several types of tissues: blood, muscle, nerve and liver cells, bone and cartilage tissues. Stem cells could be applied directly to the damaged tissue at the exact site of the damage, without drugs. For example, following a heart attack, transplanting stem cells directly at the site of the infarction has been noted to offer benefit to the outcome of the disease.

There are also strong indications but not proof yet that stem cells will be able to tackle diseases like Parkinson's, Alzheimer's, multiple sclerosis and diabetes. These diseases essentially occur when a cell type is missing, or has stopped being produced, and the stem cells "step in" to replace them. The results of stem cell treatment seem permanent. Gene therapies could correct some hereditary diseases, but can only be performed with one's own stem cells.

© *Medicare Rental and Sales*, www.medicare.ie

The actual collection of the blood isn't difficult but it will affect your decisions about whether to go with a natural third stage (no medical intervention) or a managed third stage and have the syntocinon injection. When you have a managed third stage your baby's cord must be clamped immediately. Your consultant will collect the cord blood from the umbilical cord and it doesn't cause any pain to you or your baby. All in all, the procedure takes a few minutes and you can be cuddling your newborn while it's going on. The blood is then labelled and couriered to the UK, as there are no facilities in Ireland to store the stem cells. Be sure to check with your consultant and hospital if they support this procedure; some hospitals don't. The cost is approx €1,400.

Newborn Tests and Screening

If the baby is born in an Irish hospital, it is usual to carry out screening for metabolic disorders (the Guthrie or heel prick test). If the baby is born at home, the test may be carried out by the GP or in the out-patients department of a hospital.

Guthrie Test (Heel Prick Test)

This is a routine screening test taken a few days after birth. Some experts express concern that testing for **PKU** before the baby has actually digested anything gives false information and recommend that you test your baby between one and two weeks of age. A small amount of blood is taken from your baby's heel (it's quite painful, so hold your baby yourself and nurse him right after). The blood is dropped onto a special card called the Guthrie Card and will be tested for PKU and sometimes other genetic diseases such as cystic fibrosis; ask your hospital what diseases they screen for. If you would rather not have your baby screened, you'll need to discuss this with your caregiver.

Vaccination

Most vaccinations are not given until your baby is at least two months old. However, if your baby is at risk of tuberculosis (TB) you may be offered the option of giving her a BCG shot shortly after birth.

Vaccinations given at two months, and again at four and six months, reduce the risk of diphtheria, whooping cough, Hib, tetanus and polio. Vaccinations against measles, mumps and rubella (German measles) are usually given when your baby is about a year old.

If you have concerns about possible side effects of vaccinations, discuss these with you doctor. However, it is important to stress that the risks of not vaccinating often outweigh the risks of your baby developing any side effects.

VITAMIN K

Vitamin K is routinely given in Irish hospitals. Vitamin K is mostly given so that your baby's blood will clot, and it also helps protect against a fatal disease known as newborn haemorrhagic disease, which occurs about 4–7 times per 100,000 births. Your baby will be given an intramuscular shot (usually in the thigh) of vitamin K as a precaution. Some experts feel that vitamin K is a way to ensure that any baby with haemorrhagic disease will be safe. A Japanese study showed that babies who consume 350 ml of breastmilk in the first three days following birth are protected against vitamin K deficiency. There is some dispute about the wisdom of giving high levels of vitamin K to a newborn baby, and there are also possible risks associated with the carrier substance, which has not been fully researched.

CIRCUMCISION

Circumcision of baby boys is not routinely done in Ireland, nor has it been part of our culture to circumcise babies. With the increased number of immigrants into the country and the resulting number of cross-cultural unions, it is becoming a subject that more and more Irish people are giving thought to.

Contrary to common belief, circumcision is not dictated by *any* religion. In some, such as Islam and Judaism, it is *recommended* but not mandatory.

The fact is that to circumcise the penis of a young boy is to subject him to an unnecessary operation that is, at best, extremely uncomfortable for days afterwards and, at worst, fatal. To amputate a boy's foreskin is to mutilate his genitals and serves no medical or hygienic purpose. Contrary to popular lore, a circumcised penis is not more sensitive than an uncircumcised one. The glans, which is exposed after circumcision, is not actually skin and must toughen up and de-sensitise after this operation. In fact, the foreskin is intended to protect this sensitive tip of the penis and to remove it does nobody any favours.

BREAST IS STILL BEST

If you're planning to breastfeed, it's a great idea to start learning about it before your little one arrives. There are some things you need to know that will help make breastfeeding a great experience right from the start, so let's start with some boobology. You may have gone to antenatal classes or read a few books about breastfeeding, but just like driving, reading about it or watching someone else do it isn't quite the same as doing it yourself.

As Janet Tamaro says in her book *So That's What They're For*, choosing between breastmilk and formula is like asking "Would you rather have perfectly created, safe, chemical-free organic nutritious food or IV fluid?" We can't make blood, hearts, kidneys, livers, eyes or anything else that humans need in a factory. Only human beings make the perfect parts. And only human beings make the perfect food for their babies. Think about it — how would the human race have survived for the last million years before bottles were invented?

What's so Special about Breastmilk?

The current level of breastfeeding in Ireland is still around 40 per cent; a rate which is very low in comparison to rates of 99 per cent in Norway, 96 per cent in Germany and 71 per cent in the United Kingdom. However, a Lansdowne Market Research survey into breastfeeding patterns and attitudes in Ireland in 2003 revealed that 63 per cent of Irish mothers and mothers-to-be feel that breastfeeding is better than formula feeding. It is now government policy to promote breastfeeding, and a number of initiatives have been introduced, such as "Babies Who Lunch" — welcoming and facilitating breastfeeding mothers in restaurants and hotels.

We think of formula as a good second choice. But it's not even a good third or fourth choice. Yet we are led to believe that breastmilk and formula are almost equal. You don't have to love the idea of using your breasts as your child's first refrigerator, or commit to breastfeeding your little one until he's making his first communion. Before you make up your mind not to do it, make sure it's an educated decision.

You've probably heard something along the lines of "What's wrong with formula? I was formula fed and I turned out OK!" Fair enough, but you'd be more "OK" if you'd been breastfed. Years ago, it was quite acceptable for children to bounce around the back seat of the car (and sometimes the front) with no car seats, or even seatbelts, either — and most of us did OK. But we know better now.

Studies have shown that breastfeeding lowers the risk of your baby developing the following conditions:

- Gastrointestinal and urinary tract infections;

- Lower respiratory tract illnesses;

- Otitis media;

- Bacterernia and meningitis.

Breastfeeding has also been shown to lower infant mortality and reduce the frequency of certain chronic diseases later in life (i.e. insulin dependent diabetes, Crohn's disease, ulcerative colitis and certain lymphomas). Among the benefits occurring to a mother who breastfeeds for four to six months are a lower risk of both breast and uterine cancer.

As Breastfeeding.org states, "breastfeeding provides ideal nutrition, growth hormones and infection-fighting factors which change over time as the growing infant and child's needs change; provides it inexpensively, and with no harm to the environment. Breastfed infants are healthier overall, and research is indicating that the health benefits may continue into adulthood." Virtually every woman will be able to breastfeed her infant — even those with inverted nipples and those who have had breast augmentation or reduction surgery. If breastfeeding is difficult or painful, don't give up — get help. There's lots of support out there.

SOME TRUTHS ABOUT BREASTMILK

- Breastmilk is always available, does not need mixing or sterilising and is always at the right temperature.

- Breastmilk meets all of your child's nutritional needs.

- Breastmilk will not be recalled by the manufacturer, has no "best before" date and will not harm your baby.

- Breastmilk will be a familiar taste to your baby, as it tastes like amniotic fluid, so the baby will be born liking it.

- There is no waste when you breastfeed your baby.

- Breastmilk reduces the likelihood of your child becoming obese.

- Breastmilk has more than 100 (some sources say more than 400) ingredients not found in formula, including at least four unique proteins. There are unique and powerful immune-building properties in breastmilk, and it can enhance brain development.

- Breastmilk is a living substance. Each woman's milk is individually tailored for her own baby. What's more, her milk changes constantly — both during a feed and day-by-day — to meet her baby's evolving needs. When a mother is exposed to pathogens in the environment, she produces antibodies to combat them. The mother's antibodies are then passed on to her baby via her breastmilk. (*Source*: World Alliance for Breastfeeding Action: "Breastfeeding; World Breastfeeding Week, 1997 — Nature's Way")

- Breastmilk is easier to digest than any alternative, which means less spitting up, vomiting, painful gas and colic.

- Breastmilk is the most ecological food available to humans. There is less consumption of natural resources and landfill space. The production of packaging of formula uses paper, glass, plastic and metals, all of which need to be produced and disposed of. Then there is the plastic and silicone involved in the production of the bottles and teats — not to mention the phosphates used, or water wasted, in sterilising all the equipment.

- Breastmilk can successfully be used to treat eye infections.

- Breastmilk is the *only* fluid that is not harmful if it gets into the lungs.

- Breastfeeding encourages correct growth and development of oral muscles, facial bones and promotes healthier teeth.

- Breastfeeding boosts women's self-reliance and self-esteem; by meeting the needs of their infants, they increase their confidence in their ability to parent and nurture.

- Breastfeeding protects against SIDS (cot death).

- Breastfed babies have up to 50 per cent fewer ear infections than bottle-fed babies

- Breastfeeding stimulates a mother's body to produce prolactin and oxytocin, the "mothering hormones". (Prolactin helps you feel relaxed, loving and calm. Prolactin levels can increase 10–20-fold within 30 minutes of beginning a nursing session.)

- The skin-to-skin contact offered by breastfeeding reduces the stress which babies experience when they enter the world from the warmth and safety of the womb.

- Breastfeeding enhances vaccine effectiveness.

- Breastfeeding reduces parental leave from work, as the baby is usually healthier.

- Breastfed girls have a reduced chance of suffering breast cancer in adulthood.

- Breastfeeding increases your oxytocin levels which help your uterus to contract to expel the placenta after birth.

© *www.parentingweb.com. Adapted and reproduced with kind permission.*

TIPS FOR SUCCESS

Get your baby to the breast as soon as possible — immediately if you can. Even though it doesn't seem much, colostrum is all your baby needs for the first few days, until your milk "comes in"; he's not thirsty and he's not very hungry. (You may have noticed that your breasts leaked a little in the last few weeks before birth: this is **colostrum**. This "liquid gold" is highly concentrated with nutrients and antibodies to nourish and protect your newborn).

Newborns are usually alert for about an hour after birth (some babies may be drowsy from the epidural, if you have had one). Take advantage of this time, as your baby will be very interested in your breast. Put it in your birth plan that this is very important to you. Make sure your baby isn't routinely taken away for observation, unless there is a real medical need. Try to keep your baby with you; being separated from you is upsetting. After all, he's been with you his whole life. Don't let friends or relatives talk you into sending your baby off to the nursery so you can get some rest. As tired as you are, your baby needs you. If you need help with the latch (attaching your baby to the breast properly so that it doesn't hurt), ask to see the hospital lactation consultant or your midwife. When you get home, contact the La Leche League for help or a private lactation consultant. Not all public health nurses have the experience needed to help a new mum with a breastfeeding problem.

I remember watching an amazing documentary from Sweden in which a newborn baby, less than an hour old, actually crawls to the nipple of his mother with no assistance at all — sensing her breast-milk by smell.

Within a few days of giving birth, you may well wake up in the middle of the night with two hot bowling balls instead of breasts (hot being the temperature, and it's bloody uncomfortable). This often happens when your milk comes in initially. The great news is that it's easy to fix and only temporary. An easy way to help with engorgement is first of all for Dad to take the baby and you take a warm shower or get a nice warm moist towel and gently massage your breasts and the milk will begin to flow and release some of the pressure. Then, as soon as you can, get baby on the breast for his first big meal.

Don't be alarmed if your baby seems to be constantly on the breast for the first three or four days. This does not mean the baby isn't getting enough — on the contrary, it means that the baby is so well satisfied with what you are producing for her that she can't stay away! Hungry babies cry — if your baby is constantly suckling but does not seem to be upset or distressed, then she is not hungry.

How do I know if she is getting enough milk?

Wouldn't it be so much easier if our babies came with a fluid indicator, like the petrol gauge in your car? Well it's actually simple physics — you can measure your baby's input by his output! Your baby may have only one or two wet nappies during the first day or two after birth. On about the third or fourth day, she will have at least five or six really wet nappies (six to eight if you're using cloth). A week later, 8–12 wet nappies is the norm.

The Scoop on Poop

Meconium, the greenish-black, tarry first stool, will be passed by the baby in the first day or two. (Colostrum is a natural laxative, and will help with the passing of this first stool.) Your baby will begin to have between three and five bowel movements a day, starting on or about the third day after birth. Breastfed babies tend to have yellow mustardy poops that don't smell, because breastmilk is easily digested. Breastfed babies are more "regular" than formula-fed babies. For the first year of his life, my son pooped to a schedule; we could almost time it.

During the first three or four days after birth, your baby may lose up to seven per cent of her birth weight. Once your milk supply becomes more plentiful on the third or fourth day, she will start to gain. Generally, babies gain 170g (6oz) per week. Be sure to count weight gain from the lowest weight (i.e. the baby's weight on the third or fourth day), not from birth weight.

The best way of knowing if your baby is getting enough is that she will be obviously healthy, her skin will be firm and of a healthy colour, she will be filling out and growing in length and head circumference. She will be alert and active.

If you experience any pain or discomfort when breastfeeding, or if you have any worries about your supply, please seek help immediately. Your local branch of La Leche League is an excellent form of mother-to-mother support and you may even be lucky to find a lactation consultant either through a maternity hospital or independently.

BREASTFEEDING IN THE LONGER TERM

Duration of Breastfeeding

The World Health Organisation recommends breastfeeding exclusively for the first six months; that breastmilk be the main source of food for the first twelve months; and that breastfeeding continue for at least the first two years and thereafter as long as the mother and child desire. While that might seem like an awfully long time, bear in mind that, as a baby gets older, she will not nurse as frequently, or for as long, as a newborn baby. Most toddler nurslings will only breastfeed first thing in the morning, last thing at night and perhaps on one or two other occasions during the day. Play it by ear and see what suits you and your baby. Breastmilk is liquid love and the more of it you can give your baby the better.

For guidelines on your rights as a breastfeeding mother in employment, see Appendix B, pages 227–228.

The Milk Bank

If your supply is plentiful, you might consider donating your spare milk to the milk bank. The milk bank is a place where human milk is collected, processed and stored. This milk is made available to sick babies in hospitals and other specialist baby units throughout Ireland. By donating milk to the bank you are helping tiny, premature, sick babies survive and leave hospital more quickly. For further information, contact the milk bank directly at (048) 68628333 or e-mail milkbank@sperrinlakeland.freeserve.co.uk.

BREASTFEEDING SUPPORT

If you find breastfeeding difficult, there are many people who can help and reassure you:

- *At the Hospital or at Home.* The midwife will have had much experience with breastfeeding mothers and will be able to help you get started. Some are lactation consultants and have specific training in breastfeeding support. In addition, most hospitals run a weekly drop-in breastfeeding clinic.

- *At the Local Health Centre.* Breastfeeding support groups are run by the public health nurse. Meetings take place weekly, where you and other mothers can meet the nurse to discuss any problems you might have and to seek her advice.

- *Breastfeeding Counsellors.* Cuidiu, The Irish Childbirth Trust, has a list of trained breastfeeding counsellors who will answer any queries you might have. They are available all over the country. Contact Cuidiu for the name of your nearest counsellor. In addition, the La Leche League is a voluntary group which provides information and support to women who want to breastfeed their babies. Their services include telephone counselling, monthly group meetings and a referral service to GPs and Public Health Nurses. A list of La Leche League counsellors (or "leaders") is provided in the telephone book under "La Leche League". Telephone the counsellor nearest you.

- *Breastfeeding Support Groups.* Both Cuidiu and La Leche League organise breastfeeding support groups. Contact them for the number of your nearest group. Most breastfeeding support services are available free of charge although Cuidiu and the La Leche League charge a small annual membership fee.

© *www.parentingweb.com. Adapted and reproduced with kind permission.*

KANGAROO CARE

A baby kangaroo isn't quite ready for the world when it is born but nature has devised the perfect way for the joey to thrive outside the womb with skin to skin contact with its mother. **Kangaroo care** is a way of holding a premature baby so that there is skin-to-skin contact, usually between the mother and baby — or father and baby when mum is resting. Your baby wears only a nappy, and is held upright against your bare chest. Kangaroo care has been shown to improve a premature baby's breathing and regulate his body temperature by skin-to-skin contact, and he gets the benefit of easy access to your breasts. If you give birth prematurely, check with your hospital to see if they encourage kangaroo care. Research is very supportive of this therapy.

INFANT MASSAGE

Mothers in other cultures massage their babies regularly. It is a wonderful way of connecting with your baby, helping him to adjust to life outside the womb while also lowering your own stress levels. It's a lovely routine to get into after bathtime and can help your baby sleep better (don't we all sleep better after a nice massage!).

According to wwwhomebirth.ie, the benefits of infant massage include:

- Helps the parents and baby bond;
- You become more confident handling your baby and reading his cues (non-verbal communication);
- It's a great way for Dads to connect with their baby in the evenings if they've been gone all day.

For the baby the benefits are numerous; it helps with:

- Digestion
- The circulatory system
- It calms and relaxes your baby.

There are several books about baby massage but for some taking a class is helpful, and you'll get to meet other mums. During the class the instructor demonstrates the movements to the class on a doll, with each parent following along massaging their own baby.

Infant massage is fun and enjoyable for both parent and baby. You can massage your baby from a very early age; there is now evidence that shows that sick or premature babies benefit from "touch" massage. (McClure, 1998).

TAKING CARE OF YOURSELF AFTER THE BIRTH

In an ideal world, your partner would be a teacher (a well-paid one) and you would give birth a week after the school summer holidays started. Then you and your new family would have two picture-perfect sun-filled months together, bonding and cooing over each other. Well, for those of us who aren't so lucky, the realities of those first few days and weeks can be the stuff that nightmares are made of.

Coming home with your newborn (especially if this is your first) is an exciting but terrifying trip. First of all, you can't quite believe that they are letting you leave with this little baby; you are half-expecting an alarm to go off as you walk out the hospital doors. You find yourself driving like a learner again and all of a sudden everyone else on the road is an irresponsible driver.

 The first thing to do when you get home? Get into your pjs and go to bed with your baby. Let everyone know that you're dying to show off your baby but you'd only like to have visitors in the evening/morning (whatever suits you). It's your partner's job for the next few days while you're off to make sure that you do nothing more than snuggle in bed and feed your baby. If your partner isn't Jamie Oliver, then make up a few casseroles in the run-up to your due date and freeze them so you have instant home-cooked meals at the ready.

YOUR BODY

You've escaped having periods for nine months; after birth, you'll make up for that with about six weeks of what's known as lochia (a bloody discharge) that will go on for a few weeks. It'll start off bright red and eventually turn brown, and then yellow. You won't want to look at tampons, so stick with the heavy duty pads with wings or maternity pads.

If you've had an episiotomy or have a tear (with or without stitches), whatever you do don't even think of getting a mirror out for at least a week. You won't recognise your privates, so best to remember them as they were! A few times a day, put a little warm water in the tub or into a basin and sit in it; it will help with healing and feels wonderful. Homeopathic arnica (taken orally) is reported (by mothers, not research) to be really helpful in reducing swelling.

Sometimes the extra pressure in the pelvic area combined with a long second stage of labour (pushing) can result in piles (haemorrhoids) — another good reason to leave the mirror in your makeup bag for at least a week. The good news is they will get better . . . eventually.

It will take a few weeks before you get into a routine with your baby. Don't expect everything to fall into place immediately. You're getting to know your baby and your baby is getting to know you. Take any and all offers of help! Sleep when your baby sleeps. Don't fall into the trap of trying to get caught up on cleaning the house or doing laundry. There will always be clothes to wash and plates to clean but these precious days with your new baby won't last forever. Enjoy them!

YOUR EMOTIONS

The kind of birth you have and your feelings about it will affect your transition to parenthood either positively or negatively. It can also affect breastfeeding. So often we hear, usually from well-meaning friends, that the birth experience doesn't really matter and are told "just be grateful you have a healthy baby". But that doesn't help if you didn't have the experience you were expecting. If you or a mother you know is having a hard time dealing with a birth experience, encourage them to talk about it or write down their birth story.

Sometimes being at home with a newborn all day can be isolating, especially if you don't have much family around and all your friends are at work. Check you local community centre for mother and baby gatherings or contact Cuidiu for mum and baby groups near you.

POSTNATAL DEPRESSION

Most women experience what's known as the Baby Blues during the first few days after a birth. Your hormone levels are plummeting and you've just been through the most emotional experience of your life. Sometimes, however, the "blues" become more intense and don't disappear after the early weeks of being a new mum.

Postnatal depression, like ordinary depression, is not always easy to detect, and is difficult to distinguish from the "baby blues", which will usually dissipate over time. Usually, some or all of the following symptoms will persist for at least two weeks in PND:

- Mood swings;

- "Weepiness" and generally "low" feelings;

- Feeling like you're not cut out to be a mother;

- Poor self-esteem and self-image;

- Lack of appetite or, conversely, comfort eating;

- Recurrent thoughts about self-harm, death or suicide;

- Detachment from reality;

- Inability to connect emotionally with family, especially the new baby.

Discovery Home and Health (www.discoveryhealth.co.uk) states that the risk of becoming depressed within five weeks of delivery is three times greater than the risk of depression in the general population. It can happen to any woman who has had a baby, and certain things are known to make it more likely:

- A difficult, traumatic delivery;

- Difficult home relationships;

- Lack of social support;

- Adverse life events;

- A past history of depression or postnatal depression.

PREVENTING AND COPING WITH PND

We don't know enough about PND to prevent it in the first place, but certain principles make sense.

Before the birth:

- Do make friends with other couples who are expecting or have just had a baby; among other things it makes life easier when you know that other couples are trying to adjust to parenthood just like you are;

- Don't try to be a superwoman. Having a baby may be a full-time occupation, so try to reduce commitments during your pregnancy. (If you are at work, make sure you get regular and sufficient nourishment and put your feet up during the lunch hour.)

- Do identify someone in whom you can confide. It helps so much to have a close friend you can turn to. (If you can't easily find someone, try the PND Association of Ireland, or Cuidiu, The Irish Childbirth Trust; their local groups are very supportive before and after childbirth.)

- Don't move house (if you can help it) while you are pregnant or until the baby is six months old.

- Do go to antenatal classes — and take your partner with you!

If you have suffered from PND before, that doesn't mean that you will do so again. However, it is only sensible to keep in touch with your GP (and, after the birth, your Health Visitor) so that, should there be any signs of recurrence, treatment can start at once.

After the baby has arrived:

- Do take every opportunity to get your head down. Try to learn the knack of cat-napping. Your partner can give the baby a bottle-feed at night, using your own expressed milk if you like. (If you're breastfeeding, try not to introduce a bottle for about six weeks to avoid nipple confusion.)

- Don't blame yourself or him: life is tough at this time, and tiredness and irritability on both sides can lead to quarrels. But "having a go" at each other may weaken your relationship when it needs to be at its strongest.

- Do get enough nourishment. Healthy foods like salads, fresh vegetables, fruit, fruit juices, milk and cereals are all nice, packed with vitamins and don't need much cooking.

- Don't be afraid to ask for help.

- Do find the time to have fun with your partner. Try to find a baby-sitter and get out together for a meal, a show, to see friends or just visit the pub.

- Do let yourself and your partner be intimate, even if you don't yet feel like sex: at least kiss and cuddle. This will comfort you both and lead all the sooner to the return of full sexual feeling.

Finally even if the PND is well established by the time it is recognised, support, counselling and medication will often make a big difference and will speed up eventual recovery: It's never too late!

How partners/family/friends can help

For family and friends:

- Encourage the depressed mother to seek help from a GP, public health nurse or counsellor.

- Encourage her to join a support group. Social isolation can contribute to postnatal depression.

- Try to be patient.

- Assist in arranging practical child care.

- Try to let her express her true feelings and treat them with sympathy.

- Try to find out more about postnatal depression.

Especially for fathers:

- Try, as a couple, to go out without the children, but don't force her to do anything she doesn't feel ready for.

- Frequently assure her that her illness is temporary and that she will get well.

- Encourage activity, even though she might resist, e.g. you might suggest going for a walk together.

- Try to ensure that your partner gets enough food and rest.

- Give her a massage — this will help her relax and restore her well-being.

- Reassure her of your support and that you will not abandon her.

Postnatal depression threatens the mother's and father's health, marriage, friendship and career, as well as the baby's welfare. Dealing with issues on a day to day basis can be a special challenge for family and friends. With your support and patience you can assist the depressed mother's recovery.

© Reproduced with kind permission of the PND Association of Ireland and the Royal Association of Psychiatrists in the UK.

WHAT YOUR PARENTS NEVER WARNED YOU ABOUT BECOMING PARENTS

Most expectant couples will spend countless hours in antenatal classes learning all about labour and birth; then there's the yoga class; the breastfeeding class; and then newborn basics. By the time the big day arrives, most couples are just ready to get the show on the road, give up all these classes and get on with the real business of having their baby. But as more seasoned parents will tell you, it's only after birth that the real "labour" starts. You've probably seen that all-knowing smug smile creep across your mother-in-law's face when you tell her how tired you and your partner are from a day of shopping for the nursery. You probably only figured out what that look meant six months after your baby was born — or else just reading this chapter is giving you an Oprah "aha" moment — *so that's what she was so smug about. . . .*

WHY DO BABIES CRY?

For first-time parents, changing the nappies and giving your baby a bath come relatively easy once someone has shown you how. But with smaller families and siblings living further away from each other than ever, many of us never get to hold a newborn before we hold our own. As for calming a crying baby, sometimes it's not as easy as it looks. We've come to believe that it's our fate and even a parenting rite of passage that we have to endure spates of endless crying.

Babies cry for more reasons than I can include here. It's their way of communicating, and the most common reasons are that they are hungry, wet, tired, sick, or they just need a cuddle.

In 1962, Dr T. Berry Brazelton asked 82 new mothers to record how much their normal healthy babies cried each day during the first three months of life. Dr Brazelton discovered that at two weeks of age, 25 per cent of the babies cried for more than two hours each day. By six weeks, 25 per cent cried for more than three hours a day. Reassuringly, he found that by three months almost all were back to crying for about one hour a day. (*Source:* Dr Harvey Karp, *The Happiest Baby on the Block*)

Sometimes your baby may be diagnosed with "**colic**". A colicky baby will easily fit the following "profile": he will cry for three hours a day (usually evening); three days a week; three weeks in a row. It usually starts around two weeks of age and peaks at six weeks and is often much worse in the evening. Babies are healthy and happy between crying bouts.

While many experts have tried to find a pattern to this problem, there are no consistent links between the colic and a baby's gender, prematurity, or food. There are lots of theories about why some babies tend to be more colicky than others but none really hold true when investigated thoroughly. Most parents of colicky babies share similar experiences of their infants writhing and grunting, not being comforted by feeding or holding, or they have a piercing cry like their baby is in severe pain.

The piercing cry of a baby immediately puts the parents' nervous systems on red alert. Your baby's cry is unique to your baby and was designed to get your attention — fast. How often are you told that you'll eventually figure out what each "cry" means? But that's little comfort to a new Mum and Dad with a screaming infant on their hands after a long day at work. Or no doubt someone has told you not to pick up your baby each time he cries or you'll spoil him. You can't spoil a baby! Ignoring a baby and letting him "cry it out" would be like leaving your car alarm screeching until the battery eventually dies! Your baby may only need to be changed — or he may need medical attention.

An Easy Way to Calm Your Baby

Dr Harvey Karp is a paediatrician and a child development specialist in Santa Monica, California. He has spent many years trying to figure out the mystery of colic and why it affects some babies and not others. Through his research he has developed an easy technique to turn even the fussiest baby into what he calls "The Happiest Baby on the Block" (www.thehappiestbaby.com). His highly successful method is based on four simple but revolutionary concepts:

- *The Fourth Trimester*: How to re-create the womblike atmosphere your newborn misses — outside the womb.

- *The Calming Reflex*: An "off switch" all babies are born with, which quickly soothes crying.

- *The 5 S's*: Five easy methods to turn on your baby's calming reflex.

- *The Cuddle Cure*: How to combine the 5 S's to calm even the most colicky baby.

Dr Karp believes that babies, especially in their first few months of life, can experience "fourth trimester" issues. Babies can have a difficult time getting used to the huge amount of stimuli present in life outside of mum's body. Their reaction to all of this is to cry and cry. The "5 S's" are:

- *Swaddling*: Tight **swaddling** provides the continuous touching and support your baby experienced while still in your womb. Other cultures have been doing this for centuries and "wear" their babies close to them. Interestingly, these same cultures don't have colic.

- *Side/stomach position*: Place your baby, *while holding her*, either on her left side to assist in digestion, or on her stomach to provide reassuring support. Once your baby is happily asleep, you can safely put her in her crib, on her back.

- *Shushing Sounds*: These sounds imitate the continual whooshing sound made by the blood flowing through arteries near the womb.

Did you know the noise level that your baby is used to in the womb is equivalent to a loud vacuum cleaner? The good news is that you don't have to ruin your appliances by running the hoover all day; instead, get a "white noise CD" which can be played over and over again. How many new parents break into a cold sweat when the doorbell rings after spending the last hour trying to put the baby down for his nap? I know I was almost psychotic — and my dogs would bark at the breeze! Babies are used to noise, so trying to soundproof his room to the noises of daily life (which he's used to listening to anyway) will just stress you out even more.

- *Swinging*: Newborns are used to the swinging motions that were present when they were still in your womb. Every step you took, every movement, caused a swinging motion for your baby. After your baby is born, this calming motion, which was so comforting and familiar, is abruptly gone. Your baby misses the motion and has a difficult time getting used to it not being there. Using a sling is ideal.

- *Sucking*: "Sucking has its effects deep within the nervous system," notes Karp, "and triggers the calming reflex and releases natural chemicals within the brain." This "S" can be accomplished easiest with the breast but a bottle or soother or even a finger will work too.

Not every baby will need all five techniques. Calmer babies will need only a few; fussier babies will need all of them. Gauge your success in calming your little one according to your baby's intensity. Like any other skill, it takes practice — my husband and I practised swaddling on a stuffed toy, and had it down to a fine art by the time Jack arrived. Dr Karp's Cuddle Cure may help make those first few weeks of new parenthood enjoyable instead of spending it desperately waiting to see that light at the end of the tunnel that everyone keeps talking about while you wish away those first fantastic weeks with your newborn. For more information visit www.thehappiestbaby.com.

Helping Toddlers Adjust to a New Baby

So you've sailed through the birth and now you're home with the new addition to your family. You've just settled down on the couch for a feed and your toddler looks up at you and asks, "When are we bringing the baby back?"

"We were so excited about the new baby that we didn't include Alex, our two-year-old, as much as we should — big mistake," says Gwen. "Within days of arriving home from the hospital, Alex had gone from sleeping through the night to screaming for hours and shoving our new addition Sophie whenever I tried to breastfeed. After the first day home Alex kept asking us when the new baby was going 'back' to the hospital. It was a difficult transition for all of us. I wish we had spent more time with Alex before Sophie's birth, preparing him for the changes."

Tips to Prepare your Toddler

A new baby into the family is often the first major "trauma" that a young child experiences, especially a first and previously only child. This is a whole new world for him. Suddenly he's not the centre of attention anymore; someone cuter has come along and your toddler can't get a look in! For many toddlers acting the maggot may be enough to command your attention but in some cases a resentful toddler can resort to pinching or "cuddling" the baby a little too tightly — around the neck!

Your toddler's view of the world is fairly limited; he hasn't got a lot of life experience to measure this situation by so naturally his nose is going to be a little out of joint. Up until this morning he was IT; and in the space of a few hours (in his mind), his whole life has turned upside down. He didn't ask for this new baby and doesn't understand why you can't just "take it back". Time and patience is needed to restore his sense of security, which is the reason many young kids revert in their behaviour (start wetting the bed, ask for a bottle, thumb-sucking).

- Talk to your toddler about the new baby coming. Make it something for him to look forward to. Let him listen to your tummy and talk to the baby.

- Talk about all the things he'll be able to do as a big brother and how he will be able to help you with the baby.

- Tell your toddler that the new baby is going to bring a special present for him when he gets here. (Daddy, don't forget to go and buy it beforehand!)

- Try not to disrupt his routine with lots of changes all at once. If your toddler is getting close to being moved to his "big" bed, do it well before your new baby arrives.

© Dr Amy Feldman; reproduced with kind permission.

PARENTING STYLES

Will you Ferberize or Ford your baby? No, they're not the kind of car your baby prefers, but parenting styles. These days there are as many books on parenting styles as there are birth books, and just like your pregnancy everyone has an opinion on how to do it "the right way" (i.e., their way). There are several "trendy" styles of early parenting and I don't want to recommend one over the other because parenting is such a unique and individual experience. You will probably read a number of parenting books; some of the recommendations will sit well with you and some won't, but I can guarantee that your baby hasn't read them and won't know if you're doing "it" right or not. Follow your instincts and do what works for you and your baby.

Popular styles of early parenting include:

- *"Ferberizing"*: Recommends letting your baby to "cry it out" so he learns to put himself to sleep alone.

- *"Fording"*: Recommends putting your baby on a strict schedule for feeding, napping, etc. (based on Gina Ford's *The Contented Little Baby Book*).

- *Attachment parenting*: "Wearing" your baby, sleeping with your baby, breastfeeding and generally following your instincts and your baby's cues.

If, at any time, you find yourself overwhelmed by the task of parenting, don't be afraid to seek help. Among those who can help are Parentline and Gingerbread.

THE EVOLUTION OF A MOTHER

Your Clothes

- 1st baby: You begin wearing maternity clothes as soon as your doctor confirms your pregnancy.

- 2nd baby: You wear your regular clothes for as long as possible.

- 3rd baby: Your maternity clothes *are* your regular clothes.

The Baby's Name

- 1st baby: You pore over baby-name books and practise pronouncing and writing combinations of all your favourites.

- 2nd baby: Someone has to name his or her kid after your great-aunt Mavis, right? It might as well be you.

- 3rd baby: You open a name book, close your eyes, and see where your finger points.

Preparing for the Birth

- 1st baby: You practise your breathing religiously.

- 2nd baby: You don't bother practising because you remember that last time, breathing didn't do a thing.

- 3rd baby: You ask for an epidural in your eighth month.

Your Baby's Clothes

- 1st baby: You pre-wash your newborn's clothes, colour-coordinate them, and fold them neatly in the baby's little bureau.

- 2nd baby: You check to make sure that the clothes are clean and discard only the ones the darkest stains.

- 3rd baby: Boys can wear pink, can't they?

Worries

- 1st baby: At the first sign of distress — a whimper, a frown — you pick up the baby.

- 2nd baby: You pick the baby up when her wails threaten to wake your firstborn.

- 3rd baby: You teach your three-year-old how to rewind the mechanical swing.

Activities

- 1st baby: You take your infant to Baby Gymnastics, Baby Swing, and Baby Story Hour.

- 2nd baby: You take your infant to Baby Gymnastics.

- 3rd baby: You take your infant to the supermarket and the dry cleaner.

Going Out

- 1st baby: The first time you leave your baby with a babysitter, you call home five times.

- 2nd baby: Just before you walk out the door, you remember to leave a number where you can be reached.

- 3rd baby: You leave instructions for the babysitter to call only if she sees blood.

> *At Home*
>
> - 1st baby: You spend a good bit of every day just gazing at the baby.
>
> - 2nd baby: You spend a bit of every day watching to be sure your older child isn't squeezing, poking, or hitting the baby.
>
> - 3rd baby: You spend a little bit of every day hiding from the children.

AND FINALLY . . .

Pregnancy and birth are huge events in our lives and naturally bring with them questions and doubts. During those nine months all we seem to hear in our heads every day are those "What ifs?" — so let's look at them from a slightly different angle.

What If?

- What if I have an easy labour and my baby has a wonderful, gentle birth?

- What if everything happens just as I hoped it would?

- What if I breastfeed easily?

- What if having a baby is the most empowering experience of my life and I relish every moment of it?

APPENDIX A: GUIDE TO MATERNITY UNITS IN IRELAND

The following information was provided by Cuidiu from their Annual Maternity Hospital Review for 2003. Each year, hospitals are invited to submit their birth statistics; not all maternity units choose to participate. Some only provided information for 2002. Due to lack of participation, the guide was not completed for 2005. All figures are for 2003, except where stated.

I encourage you to read through the various hospital submissions and not just the hospital you are planning to attend. This will give you a better idea of what's going on throughout the country. Some hospitals provided more information than others, so they aren't all easily comparable. Note how many hospitals are even close to the World Health Organisation recommended rates for caesarean section (15 per cent). You will also see considerably high rates of inductions and episiotomies. Hospitals also have different protocols for administering Vitamin K.

ROTUNDA HOSPITAL, DUBLIN

No. of Births	Ventouse/ Forceps	Induction	Failed Inductions for primips	Episiotomy	Caesarean Section
6,731	16.5%	19%	39.5%	16.8%	26.6%*

Note: figures are for 2004. * Reduced from 28.2% in 2003.

Coombe Hospital, Dublin

Statistics

No. of Births	Caesarean Section	Induction rate	Episiotomies	
			Primips	*Multips*
8,409	24%	25%	21%	5.3%

National Maternity Hospital, Dublin

Statistics

No. of Births	Caesarean Section (2004)	C-Section: Method of Analgesia		
		Spinal	*Epidural*	*General Anaesthetic*
8,022	17%	54%	33%	13%

Rates:	Epidural	Induction	Labour Accelerated	Foetal Monitoring	Episiotomy
Primips	63%	22%	55%	68%	38.9%
Multips	38%	19%	11%	27%	9%

Rates:	Ventouse	Forceps	Vaginal Breech Deliveries	Vaginal Deliveries of Twins
Primips	14.9%	6%	14.5%	55%
Multips	4%	1%	23%	67%

Labour

- Birth plans need to be discussed with the care provider antenatally
- Routine rupture of membranes
- Mobility encouraged
- Criteria for inducing labour: any condition that may put infant or mother at risk.

Delivery

- The mother is free to choose her own position for labour and birth
- Birthing balls, beanbags and mats are available
- Syntometrine is now given routinely, natural 3rd stage on request

- Breastfeeding and "skin-to-skin contact" encouraged for all babies
- Assistance for mothers wishing to breastfeed is offered to commence breastfeeding as soon as possible.

Postnatal Ward

- Vitamin K given to all babies with consent
- BCG vaccinations: Mondays, Wednesdays, Thursdays; baby over 24-hours-old
- Baby stays with mother all the time ('Rooming-in' is policy for all mothers and babies)
- Baby Care Rooms in all wards
- PKU/heel prick test is the only routine test performed on baby
- Supplementing breastfed babies: babies are supplemented if medically indicated.

Length of stay

- Primips: 2–3 days
- Multip: 2 days
- Caesarean section: 5 days

Postnatal Period

- Mothers may telephone up to six weeks
- Emergency phone numbers given on discharge
- Baby clinic: by appt only referred by neonatologist or SCBU
- Referral of all mothers to PHN; liaison PHN clerk
- Breastfeeding support services: special clinic on Fridays 10.00–12.00
- Postnatal exercise classes offered by physios: Mondays, Wednesdays, Fridays, 10.30am
- Postnatal baby care classes organised in hospital: Tuesdays and Thursdays, 10.30am
- Postnatal baby massage for babies over six weeks by appointment

ERINVILLE, CORK

Statistics

| No. of Births | Caesarean Section | Induction rate | Episiotomies | |
			Primips	Multips
3,053	27.1%	25.6%	n/a	n/a

Vacuum Delivery Rate	Forceps Delivery Rate	Vaginal Breech Delivery Rate	Multiple Births	Vaginal Delivery of Twins
14.1%	3.5%	n/a	37	n/a

No. of maternity beds:

Public	Semi-private	Private
34	18	4

Labour

- Accommodation: three two-bedded rooms
- Birth companion (1) is welcome at all times
- Birth plans are facilitated
- Foetal monitoring done routinely on admission
- No shave
- No enema
- Midwife is assigned to every mother
- Mobility is encouraged
- Mother may take fruit juice and water in labour
- 24-hour epidural service.
- Other pain relief: Psycho prophylaxis, Entonox, Pethidine and TENS.
- Foetal monitoring by **Pinard** stethoscope and **cardiotogography**.

Birth

- Mother gives birth in the same room in which she was during labour
- Birthing beds available
- Partner/companion welcome to stay throughout all births including caesarean section

- Where a parent has a disability or language difficulty we facilitate by giving whatever is required; extra support people are most welcome, e.g. interpreter/sign language
- The mother is free to choose her own position for birth
- **Lithotomy** position is used for instrumental delivery, breech and also for suturing.
- The cord is cut at birth or, if the baby is in good condition, when it stops pulsating
- Natural management of the third stage on request
- Baby stays with the mother at all times.

Neonatal Unit

- 10 neonatal intensive care cots
- 2 full time consultant neonatologists
- Parents may visit at all times; visiting extended to grandparents only; siblings may visit at the discretion of the midwife on duty
- There is a room available for parents to stay in emergency circumstances; hot refreshments available 24 hours a day
- Kangaroo care is practised
- Breastfeeding is encouraged on demand
- If the mother of a breastfeeding baby is discharged before her baby special arrangements are made to support her continuing to breastfeed
- Mothers are encouraged to spend as much time as possible with baby
- Breast pumps are available for use in the unit
- Containers for breast milk are supplied and freezer is available
- Use of teats is utilised as little as possible and feeds are timed so that mothers can feed as much as possible
- Mother's own milk or formula is used to supplement or complement. But formula is only given to breastfeeding babies where mother's own milk is not available and at the request and consent of the mother
- 90% of the babies in the unit are breastfed

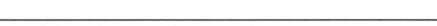

- Methods of topping up or complementing feeds are tube, teat and syringe
- Neonatal individualised developmental care is practised.

Postnatal care

- Vitamin K is given to all babies orally
- BCG is not given in the hospital
- Heel prick test and hip check is done routinely
- Blood sugars are not done routinely
- Baby remains with mother at all times
- Rooming-in policy in the hospital. (Unified Maternity Services encourages rooming-in. No matter how you choose to feed your baby, you are encouraged to remain with your baby 24 hours a day. All babies should stay with their mothers unless they are separated for medical reasons, for example if your baby is admitted to the Baby Unit.)
- Breastfeeding is encouraged on demand
- Breastfed babies are not supplemented routinely. If a mother wants her baby to be supplemented, she will discuss this with the midwife and it will be documented in her chart
- Visiting hours 3.00 to 4.00 pm and 7.00 to 8.30 pm; open visiting for husbands/partners only
- 60% of mothers initiate breastfeeding
- 58% breastfeed on discharge
- Mothers may telephone the hospital at any time if they have any queries
- Breastfeeding support available by phone or through support group every Tuesday morning in the Erinville from 10.00 to 12.00 or in St Finbars on Thursday afternoons from 2.00 to 4.00 pm
- Mothers and babies have postnatal check at six weeks with their GP
- Every mother is referred to the Public Health Nurse
- Every mother is referred to her GP.

Special Needs or Circumstances

- Wheelchair accessible, including the toilet on every ward

- Wheelchair parking available
- Women with communication difficulties communicate through their partner or interpreter
- Interpreter service is available
- Special support available for parents in the case of stillbirth or miscarriage
- Bereavement counselling available

LETTERKENNY MATERNITY UNIT, DONEGAL

Statistics

No. of Births	Epidural Rate	Caesarean Section	C-Section under Spinal/Epidural
1,758	12.1%	21.8%	14.4%

Rates:	Induction	Labour Accelerated	Episiotomy	Ventouse	Forceps
Primips	10.2%	14.7%	12.8%	7.1%	0.8%
Multips	11.6%	6.6%	6%	2%	0.1%

Rates:	Vaginal Breech Deliveries	Vaginal Deliveries of Twins
Primips	0.2%	0.1%
Multips	0.1%	0.2%

No. of maternity beds:

Public	Semi-private	Private
30	6	4

Number of Obstetricians: 3

Antenatal Care

- Referral letter required from GP
- Clinic times 9.00 am to 1.00 pm / 1.00 pm to 5.00 pm
- There is an appointment system

- Mothers opt for either combined care or private care
- Midwives booking/consultation at all clinics
- Consultation with antenatal education co-ordinator at clinics
- Continuity of care: seen by consultant 1st visit; care then shared with registrar/midwife
- Information packs given to all on 1st visit (Breast Feeding, Rooming In, Skin to Skin, Health Education, etc.)
- All mothers scanned for dates on 1st visit (visit from 18–22 weeks)
- Breech presentation, multiple pregnancy: each consultant decides on management.

Labour

- Accommodation: 1 four-bedded first stage room, 3 single delivery rooms
- Birth companion (1; can change during labour if wishes) welcome at all times
- Birth plans facilitated
- Admission CTG carried out, continuous monitoring in labour only on high risk, intermittent **auscultation** for low risk
- Normal labour — no intervention
- Mobilisation in labour encouraged
- Access to bath in labour if required
- Mother may take light diet, fluids in early labour
- Criteria for inducing labour: assessed individually
- Epidural service on offer 24 hours
- Other forms of pain relief available: Entonox, Pethidine, TENS, and Reflexology
- Foetal Monitoring: **Pinards**; **Sonicaid**; Cardiotocography.

Delivery

- Mothers deliver in single delivery room
- Partners/companion welcome to stay throughout all deliveries.
- Birthing bed available

- The mother is encouraged to choose her own position for delivery (if circumstances permit)
- May deliver on mattress on floor
- Birthing ball available
- Lithotomy position used for instrumental deliveries and suturing
- Cord cut depending on midwives' practice by midwife or doctor
- Active management practised routinely but natural third stage management is permitted on request
- Skin-to-Skin practised at all deliveries, including caesareans; partners included.

Special Care Unit

- 2 Intensive care cots
- 5 Special care cots
- 3 Full-time consultant paediatricians
- Parents have free access to their baby
- Other family members by arrangement
- Family room available
- Mothers can breastfeed on demand
- Storage facilities for breastmilk available
- Methods: spoon, syringe, tube and bottle.

Postnatal ward

- Vitamin K given to all babies with written consent
- BCG offered in the hospital
- Routine tests on babies PKU, Beutler
- Rooming-in practised
- Mothers encouraged to breastfeed on demand
- Extended meal times to facilitate feeding
- Visiting: afternoons and evenings — strictly no visiting 1.00 pm to 2.00 pm rest period
- Children allowed to visit.

Length of Stay

- Primips 4/5 Days
- Multips 2/3 Days
- C-sections 5 Days.

Breastfeeding

- 42% mothers initiate breast feeding
- 33.8% discharged breast feeding
- Breastfeeding drop in clinic every Thursday pm.
- Telephone advice if required
- Discharged under care of Public Health Nurse.

Special Needs

- Wheelchair accessible including toilet facilities on all floors
- Communication difficulties: hospital has leaflets and booklets in braille
- Interpreters available for non-nationals
- Support for parents in case of stillbirth or miscarriage
- Pregnancy Loss Clinic
- Bereavement counselling available
- Opportunity to return to hospital to discuss with relevant consultant/midwifery staff.

MAYO GENERAL HOSPITAL, CASTLEBAR

Statistics

No. of Births (2002)	Epidural Rate	Induction Rate	Accelerated Labour	Caesarean Section	Episiotomy Rate
1,426	31.6%	26.5%	24.6%	18.2%	22%

No of Obstetricians: 2 permanent and 2 job sharing

No. of multiple births in the last 5 years: 78 sets of twins; 2 sets of triplets

Our Lady of Lourdes, Drogheda

Statistics

No. of Births (2002)	Epidural Rate	Caesarean Section	VBAC	Induction Rate	Labour Accelerated
3,255	28%	25%	40%	26%	25%

Episiotomy		Ventouse	Forceps	Vaginal Breech Delivery	Vaginal Delivery of Twins
Primips	Multips				
26%	1%	11.1%	3.5%	0.4%	55%

No. of maternity beds:

Public	Semi-private	Private
30	15	10

Number of Obstetricians: 6

No. of multiple births in the last 5 years: Twins, 199; Triplets, 6

Antenatal care

- Referral letter needed from GP
- Appointment system is in place
- Midwives' couch available during some consultant-led antenatal clinics for women who are deemed "low risk"
- Continuity of care: mothers attend the same consultant's team for the duration of the pregnancy. If a woman is attending the midwives' couch, she will usually see the same midwife at each visit
- 100% of women opt for combined antenatal care between the GP and obstetrician/hospital
- Mothers carry their own antenatal notes
- Refreshments available from the coffee shop
- Information leaflets available in the waiting areas
- Pregnancy information leaflets provided at the 1st antenatal visit
- Ultrasound: all mothers have at the first antenatal visit and subsequently during the pregnancy if indicated
- Amniocentesis is not available

- Women may be referred to the Midwifery Day Unit or to the Antenatal Ward for assessment during pregnancy
- Outreach antenatal clinics: Louth County Hospital Dundalk; Our Lady's Hospital Navan, Co Meath.

Labour
- Accommodation: 6 single rooms; 1 three-bedded room; 1 four-bedded room.
- Birth partner/s (1–2) welcome at all times
- Birth plans encouraged
- Midwife assigned to each mother; 1:1 care not always possible
- Routine Electronic Foetal Monitoring (CTG) on admission
- Mobility/ambulation/upright positions during labour encouraged
- Birth balls, floor mats, bean bags, wedges available
- Access to bath and/or shower (shower stool/birth ball for use in shower)
- Fluids not restricted
- Food not restricted except following administration of narcotic analgesia and for women with identified risk factors, e.g. previous C/S
- Pain relief: Epidural, TENS, Entonox, and warm water bath/showers, Pethidine
- Criteria for inducing labour: postmaturity, pre eclampsia, maternal age and infertility, foetal concern
- Continuous Electrical Foetal Monitoring: Figures not available
- Forms of foetal monitoring available: Pinard Stethoscope, Doppler, CTG
- Limited Home Birth Service within 30 mile radius of hospital in NEHB area if staff available.

Birth
- Mother gives birth in the same room in which she was in established labour
- Birth beds in all rooms
- Birth stools, floor mats, bean bags and wedges available
- Birth partner/s welcome to stay for all vaginal births

- Birth partners welcome for birth by caesarean section under regional anaesthesia
- The mother is free to choose her own position for birth. Upright positions encouraged
- Lithotomy position used for assisted vaginal deliveries — vacuum, forceps, breech
- Cord cut immediately or following cessation of pulsation at mother's request
- Active management of 3rd stage practised routinely
- Expectant management (physiological) at mother's request following normal labour
- 42% of delivery room midwives have attended WHO/UNICEF Breastfeeding Programme
- 50% of delivery room midwives have attended "Active Birth" workshops.

Neonatal Unit
- 16 cots: 3 intensive care; 2 high dependencies; 11 special care
- Isolation rooms
- Full time consultant neonatologist
- Parents have free access to the baby; siblings by arrangement and grandparents to cot side
- Kangaroo care is practised
- Rooms are available for both parents to stay overnight
- Canteen facility available if required
- Mother can feed the baby on demand
- If the mother of a breastfeeding baby is discharged before her baby, "cup feeding" is encouraged in her absence; parents' room available.
- Emphasis on parentcraft, e.g. feed demonstrations, bath, etc.
- Formula feed if breastfeeding only with mum's permission to supplement or complement.
- Alternative methods for supplementing breastfeeding: spoon, cup, syringe, tube, bottle or supplementer ("if required")
- Multiple births: information on parents support groups are provided and links with other families arranged.

- Information leaflets: parents support book unit's own, cot death, BCG/PKU, breastfeeding, immunisation information and discharge advice given.

Postnatal Ward

- Rooming-in is practised within the unit
- Infant security tagging is in place
- Vitamin K is given to all babies following oral consent from mothers
- BCG vaccine may be given in hospital
- No routine tests on babies except heel prick
- Breastfeeding on demand is encouraged; breastfed babies receive supplement feed only when medically indicated
- The lactation consultant will see mother post-delivery. There are 4 lactation consultants within the unit. 53% of mothers breastfeed
- Parents visit when they wish. There is no visiting during the rest period or at meal times. Rest period 13:00–15:00. Children of mothers can visit
- Physiotherapist sees each mother individually
- The services of the social work department are available
- Babies registration; Each mother is seen by the registration secretary

Length of stay

- Primip: 2–3 days
- Multips: 1–2 days
- C-sections: 4–5 days
- Six hourly discharge facility if requested.

Postnatal Period

- Mother and baby have their six-week postnatal check with their GP
- Mother may telephone the hospital for advice at any time
- All mothers and babies are referred to the Public Health Nurse
- A letter is sent out to each GP.

Special Needs

- Wheelchair access

- Toilets on the ground floor
- Communication: interpreter services available.
- Counselling: social work and pastoral care support and follow-up for families.
- All special needs are accommodated where possible.

PORTIUNCULA, BALLINASLOE

Statistics:

No. of Births (2002)	Epidural Rate		Induction Rate	Labour Accelerated	
	Primips	Multips		Primips	Multips
1,746	80%	60%	31%	35%	5%

Episiotomy		Ventouse	Forceps	Vaginal Breech Delivery	Vaginal Delivery of Twins
Primips	Multips				
30%	10%	13%	5%	0.3%	0.23%

Caesarean Section Rate	C-Section: Method of Anaesthetic	
	Spinal	General Anaesthetic
26.1%	85%	15%

No. of maternity beds:

Public	Semi-private	Private
18	7	8

Number of Obstetricians: 3

Multiple births in last 5 years: 26 sets of twins

Labour

- Accommodation: 4 single rooms
- Birth companion (1) welcome at all times including during examinations
- Birth plans facilitated
- Foetal monitoring performed routinely on admission

- No shave
- No enema
- No routine ARM
- Midwife or student midwife shared with another mother
- Walking encouraged
- Mother may take "light diet in normal cases"
- Access to bath and / or shower
- Pain relief: Epidural, Entonox, Pethidine, TENS and Acupuncture
- Criteria for inducing labour: medical and post-dates
- Forms of foetal monitoring available: Pinard, Sonicaid, CTG
- 100% of women are monitored electronically; intermittent in all cases.

Delivery
- Mother delivers in the same single room in which she was during labour
- Partner/companion welcome to stay throughout all deliveries including caesarean section
- The mother is not free to choose her own position for delivery
- Lithotomy position used for instrumental deliveries and foetal blood sampling
- Cord cut by midwife or doctor who delivers baby when pulsation ceases; father can cut cord
- Natural third stage management is permitted on request
- Vaginal deliveries after previous caesarean: permitted.

Postnatal
- Additional skilled assistance for breastfeeding mothers: Consultant Lactation Specialist
- Vitamin K injection routinely given to all babies
- No routine tests on babies except heel prick test
- Baby stays with mother all the times
- Mother can breastfeed on demand at night.

MIDLAND REGIONAL HOSPITAL, PORTLAOISE

Statistics

No. of Births (2003)	Epidural Rate	Induction Rate	Accelerated Labour	Caesarean Section	Episiotomy Rate
1,431	12%	16.02%	n/a	24%	n/a

No. of maternity beds:

Public	Private
15	8

No of Obstetricians: 3

Multiple births (for the last 5 years): 75

Labour

- Accommodation: single rooms available
- Birth companion (1) welcome at all times.
- Birth plans facilitated "as far as possible"
- Foetal monitoring done routinely on admission
- No shave
- No routine ARM
- Midwife assigned to each mother
- Walking encouraged
- Mother may take "light meals except if liquor is meconium-stained"
- Access to bath and/or shower
- Pain relief: Epidural, Entonox, Pethidine, Massage, TENS, Reflexology, Aromatherapy and warm water baths
- Criteria for inducing labour: in baby's interest, 42 weeks gestation if the cervix is ripe; reduced liquor and reduced foetal movements
- Forms of foetal monitoring available: Sonicaid; Cardiotogography.

Delivery

- Mother delivers in the same room in which she was during labour

- Partner/companion welcome to stay throughout all deliveries except caesarean section
- The mother is free to choose her own position for delivery
- Lithotomy position used for "forceps and vacuum deliveries"
- All mothers are encouraged after delivery to have 30 minutes' skin-to-skin contact with their baby
- Breastfeeding is initiated within one hour after delivery
- Cord cut by "midwife usually" after pulsation is stopped; father can participate "if he so wishes"
- Syntometrine 1 amp given after 3rd stage i.e. delivery of baby (managed third stage)
- Vaginal deliveries after previous caesarean: mother would get trial of labour. If labour does not progress at a satisfactory rate then mother would require another caesarean section.

Postnatal Ward

- Vitamin K given to all babies orally
- BCG given in the hospital on Mondays and Thursdays
- Heel prick test done routinely on babies
- Baby stays with mother all of the time
- Access to food between evening meal and breakfast: "Sandwiches at 9.00 pm".
- Visiting: No visiting after 9.00 pm. Visitors can come in during the day except at meal times — encouraged to wait in sitting room. Also when mother is breastfeeding. Children can visit.

Length of Stay

- Primips: 4 days
- Multips: 3 days
- Caesarean Section: 5 days.

St Finbarr's Unit, Cork

Statistics:

No. of Births (2002)	Induction Rate	Augmented Labour	Non-augmented Labour	Caesarean Section Rate
2,080	25%	33.7%	28.7%	20.3%

Episiotomy	Ventouse	Forceps	Vaginal Breech Delivery	Vaginal Delivery of Twins
7.8%	12.65%	1.7%	16.1%	93.3%

No. of antenatal beds:

Public	Semi-private
17	4

No. of postnatal beds:

Public	Semi-private	Private
19	6	5

Multiple births in 2002: 28 sets of twins, 2 sets of triplets

Labour

- Birth companion is welcome at all times
- Birth plans are encouraged
- Foetal Heart Monitoring by Pinard stethoscope and Cardiotogography
- Mobility is encouraged
- Women may have fruit juice/water/milk and light meal
- 24 hour Epidural service
- Other pain relief: **Psycho prophylactics**, Entonox, Tens, Pethidine.

Birth

- Recovery rooms: 2; birthing rooms: 3 (single: 2; two-bedded: 1)
- The woman gives birth in the same room in which she was during labour as far as possible

---

- Birth companions welcome to stay throughout all examinations and births including caesarean sections if the labouring woman wishes
- Where a woman has a disability or language problem we facilitate by giving whatever is required; extra support people are welcome — interpreter/sign language
- Women are encouraged to choose a position for birth that is comfortable for them
- Lithotomy position is used for vacuum, forceps or breech; it may also be used for suturing
- Natural management of the third stage of labour on request
- Cord is cut at birth unless otherwise requested, by birth attendant or father if he wishes
- Baby stays with the mother at all times
- Breastfeeding is initiated soon after birth when mother is comfortable.

Special Care Baby Unit
- There are 12 intensive care cots
- Parents may visit at all times
- Visiting extended to grandparents only; siblings may visit at the discretion of the midwife/nurse in charge
- There is a Parenting Room for emergency use or for a mother to stay with her baby prior to the baby's discharge
- Breastfeeding on demand is encouraged
- Should a breastfeeding mother be discharged prior to her baby, special arrangements are made to facilitate her continuing to breastfeed
- Breast pumps are available; containers for breast milk are supplied and a freezer is on site
- Where possible mother's own milk is used to supplement or complement
- 80–90% of babies are breastfed.

Postnatal Care
- Vitamin K is given to all babies orally
- PKU and Hip check are done routinely
- Baby remains with mother at all times; rooming-in is a hospital policy

- Breastfeeding on demand is encouraged, supplemented feeds are not given
- All babies wear a security tag whilst in hospital.

St Luke's, Kilkenny

Statistics

The statistical information is for the year 2002

No. of Births	Epidural Rate	Caesarean Section	Induction Rate	Labour Accelerated
1,592	34%	26%	11.5%	29.5%

Episiotomy	Ventouse	Forceps
18%	15.5%	1.5%

Number of Obstetricians: 3

No. of multiple births in last five years: 61 sets of twins

- Breech Presentation: advised to have a Caesarean Section
- Breastfeeding initiation: 39.5%
- Breastfeeding on discharge: 31.5%
- Special Care Baby Unit: New SCBU opened in May 2002

Length of stay

- Primips: 3 to 4 days
- Multips: 2 to 3 days
- Caesarean section: 5 days

St Munchin's, Limerick

Statistics

No. of Births (2002)	Epidural Rate	Caesarean Section	VBAC	Induction Rate	Labour Accelerated
4,396	41.53%	26.76%	n/a	28.98%	n/a

Episiotomy	Ventouse	Forceps	Vaginal Breech Delivery	Vaginal Delivery of Twins
n/a	11.1%	1.55%	0.43%	n/a

No. of maternity beds:

Public	Semi-private	Private
52	12	15

Number of Obstetricians: 6

No. of multiple births in the last 5 years: 272 sets of twins, 8 sets of triplets

Labour

- Accommodation: 1 three-bedded first stage room, 5 single rooms
- Birth companion (1) welcome at all times including examinations
- Birth plans facilitated
- Foetal monitoring done routinely on admission.
- ARM carried out "with consent"
- No shave
- No enema
- Midwife assigned to each mother — guaranteed?
- Walking encouraged
- Mother may take fluids only — usually iced water
- Access to shower
- Pain relief: Epidural, Entonox and Pethidine
- Criteria for inducing labour: post-maturity, Macrosomia (very big baby), and any other obstetric problems

- 100% of women are monitored electronically: "All mothers have admission CTG of 20 minutes and continuous foetal monitoring for obstetric problems
- Forms of foetal monitoring available: Pinard, Sonicaid, Cardiotogography.

Delivery
- Mother delivers in the same room in which she was during labour
- Birthing bed available
- Partner/companion welcome to stay throughout all deliveries including caesarean section
- The mother is free to choose her own position for delivery including giving birth on the floor
- Lithotomic position used for "forceps and ventouse deliveries and suturing"
- Cord cut by "midwife or partner if he wishes" after pulsation has stopped
- Active management practised routinely but natural third stage management is permitted on request.

Caesarean Section
- Vaginal deliveries after previous caesarean: no hospital policy
- Additional skilled assistance for breastfeeding mothers: (1) If under spinal, bonding with baby in operating theatre as soon as possible after delivery — touching, holding; (2) Breastfeeding in recovery; (3) Transfer to ward with baby in arms and partner present; (4) Recommence or commence B/F in postnatal ward. Usual time in recovery 15–20 mines.

Special Care Unit
- 21 special care cots
- Full time consultant neonatologist
- Parents, grandparents and siblings have unrestricted access to the baby
- There is a room available for parents to stay
- Mother can feed the baby on demand

- Modified version of kangaroo care is practised
- Three full-time consultant paediatricians
- Mother's own milk or formula ("only on mum's request") used to supplement or complement.
- Methods: bottle ("only on mum's request/permission must be given"), syringe, cup and tube.

Postnatal Ward
- Vitamin K given to all babies by injection
- BCG not given in the hospital
- No routine tests on babies except heel prick test
- Baby stays with mother all the time
- Mother can breastfeed on demand at night
- Breastfed babies sometimes supplemented by mother's own milk, water or formula ("cup feed of same")
- Access to food between evening meal and breakfast: "None — can have tea/coffee, toast if requested"
- Visiting: partner/parent/next of kin: 24 hours; other visitors: 2.00 pm – 4.00 pm / 7.00 pm — 9.00 pm. Children can visit.

Length of stay:
- Primips: 4 days
- Multips: 3 days
- C-Sections: 5 days.

Postnatal Period
- Mother may telephone hospital at any time if she has queries
- Emergency 24-hour service for mother and baby indefinitely
- Drop-in breastfeeding/bottle feeding clinic one afternoon a week
- Mother and baby have their GP or consultant obstetrician
- Referral to Public Health Nurse: "notification of birth".

TRALEE GENERAL HOSPITAL

Statistics

No. of Births	Ventouse	Forceps	Vaginal Breech Delivery	Vaginal Delivery of Twins
1,458	17%	3.69%	0.81%	9 sets

Rates:	Epidural	Induction	Labour Accelerated	Episiotomy	
				Vaginal Delivery	Adjusted following Instrumental Delivery
Total:	33%	30.54%	48.68%		
Primips	of which 65%	of which 48.68	n/a	39%	25.8%
Multips	of which 35%	of which 51.5%	n/a	6.8%	17.55%

Caesarean Section Rate					Anaesthetic Used		
Total	of which Primips	of which Multips	of which Elective	of which Emergency	GA	Spinal	Epid.
23.15%	45.48%	54.52%	41.57%	58.43%	47.89%	45.18%	6.93%

No. of maternity beds:

Public	Private
26	6

Number of Obstetricians: 3

Multiple Births in 2002: 24 sets of twins

Labour

- Accommodation: 4 single labour/delivery room
- Admission room / triage room: 4 beds
- 1 birth companion welcome and may stay at all times
- Birth plans facilitated
- Foetal monitoring done routinely on admission

- No shave
- No enema
- No routine ARM
- 1 midwife assigned to each mother — guaranteed?
- Walking encouraged
- Mothers may take light diet and fluids
- Access to bath and shower
- Multip breech presentation — consultant's decision
- Primip breech — elective c-section
- Pain relief: Epidural, Entonox, Pethidine, TENS and warm water baths
- Criteria for inducing labour: consultant decision
- All women are monitored electronically (routinely on admission and following induction)
- Form of foetal monitoring available: Pinard, Sonicaid and CTG

Delivery
- Mother delivers in the same room as she was when in labour
- Partner/birth companion welcome to stay throughout all normal deliveries
- Position used for delivery: 1. Left Lateral; 2. Supine; 3. Knee Chest; 4. Lithotomy position used for instrumental deliveries or perineal suturing. Mother is free to choose any of these positions for delivery
- Cord cut when pulsation has ceased. Birthing partner / father may participate if he wishes.
- Third stage management: Syntometrine given I.M. at birth of anterior shoulder.

Special Care Unit
- 10 Special Care Cots
- 2 full time paediatricians
- Parents and grandparents and siblings welcome to visit the unit
- There is no room available for parents to stay
- Dining room facilities available for parents at meal times by day and at night

- Kangaroo care is practised.
- Infant may be fed on demand where appropriate
- If the mother of a breastfeeding baby is discharged before her baby she is encouraged to attend for feed during the day and/or bring expressed breastmilk which may be stored in the unit.

Postnatal Care
- Vitamin K administered to all babies with mother's consent
- BCG not given in the hospital
- No routine blood test done on babies except PKU test. Other blood tests are done when ordered by paediatrician
- Infants stay with mother
- Majority of infants sleep in cot beside mother at night (rooming-in currently being introduced)
- Mothers are encouraged to breastfeed on demand.
- Breastfed infants supplemented with mother's expressed breastmilk or by formula at mother's request; cup feeding encouraged or teat feeds.

Length of stay:
- Primip: 4 Days
- Multip: 2/3 Days
- C-section: 5 Days

Postnatal Period
- Mother may phone the hospital at any time if she has a query
- Mother has six-week postnatal check with her GP
- Infant six-week check with GP
- Public Health Nurse informed re birth, by birth notification on discharge.
- Public Health Nurse notified by telephone re early discharge.
- Liaison Public Health Nurse visits the unit Tuesday and Friday.
- GP discharge letter, interim report on discharge.

WEXFORD MATERNITY UNIT

Statistics

No. of Births	Epidural	Caesarean Section	Induction	Episiotomy	Ventouse	Forceps
1,856	46.5%	20%	10%	11%	8.5%	2%

No. of maternity beds:

Public	Semi-private	Private
18	0	5

Number of Obstetricians: 3

No. of multiple births in the last 3 years: 44 sets of twins, 1 set of triplets

Labour

- Accommodation: 2 single rooms and 2 two-bedded rooms
- Birth plans are encouraged
- Foetal monitoring done routinely on admission (20 min) with consent of mother
- No shave/no enema
- ARM not performed routinely and done with consent of mother
- Mobilisation encouraged
- Access to bath available
- Women who are deemed low-risk are encouraged to eat high carbo-hydrate, low residue food in the latent phase of labour and fluids only in the active phase
- Midwife shared with another woman, depending on no. of women in labour
- Pain relief available: mobilisation and position changes; Epidural, TENS; Pethidine; Entonox
- Criteria for induction: post-dates or medical reason
- Forms of foetal monitoring available include: Pinard, Sonacaid and Electric Foetal Monitoring (EFM)

- All women are offered electronic foetal monitoring on admission and is performed with their consent.

Delivery
- Partner welcome to stay throughout all deliveries except caesarean section
- Birthing beds available in all delivery rooms
- Active or physiological management of third stage facilitated (as woman prefers and condition dictates)
- The woman is free to choose her own position for delivery (low-risk cases)
- Lithotomy position used for ventouse/forceps deliveries.
- With all twin deliveries we aim for vaginal delivery unless medically indicated otherwise
- Vitamin K given to all babies by injection following explanation and consent from parent
- Caesarean section: anaesthesia used: spinal
- VBAC: trial of labour offered.

Postnatal Care
- Women have a daily postnatal check performed by the midwife
- Women who have had an LSCS have their 6/52 check at the hospital
- Baby has its 6/52 check with the GP
- BCG given in hospital with consent
- Guthrie test performed on all babies with consent (PKU)
- Rooming-in is practised, i.e. baby stays with mother at all times
- Breastfeeding is encouraged and facilitated; 40% of mothers initiate breastfeeding; 35% continue to breastfeed on discharge.

Length of stay
- Primips: 2-3 days
- Multips: 1-2 days
- Caesarean sections: 5 days
- Domino: 6-24 hours.

Special Care Baby Unit

- 4 special care cots
- 2 consultant paediatricians
- Parents/grandparents and siblings have free access to visit baby
- Kangaroo care is not practised
- Breastfeeding is encouraged
- Formula is used to supplement or complement baby if medically in-dicated.

HOSPITALS IN NORTHERN IRELAND

Provided by BirthChoiceUK.com (Year 2002)

Hospital	*Induction*	*Caesarean Section*	*Instrumental/ Assisted Deliveries*
Causeway Hospital	33.1%	21.9%	8.2%
Craigavon Area Hospital	27.1%	30.1%	11.4%
Daisy Hill, Newry	31%	22.6%	9.4%
Lagan Valley Hospital	30%	21.5%	10%
Mater, Belfast	39.4%	25.7%	14%

When you've finished reading through the hospital information, go back and re-read this appendix again. You'll then be more familiar with what constitutes "mother-friendly care" — and what doesn't. Did you notice a pattern? Look at the high rates of labour inductions and accelerations, high rates of episiotomies and caesarean sections. When did birth become a frantic sprint to a finishing line that keeps being moved?

APPENDIX B:
GOVERNMENT GUIDELINES —
WHAT ARE YOUR OPTIONS?

CARE OPTIONS

Depending on whether you have private health insurance, you may choose to sign up as a *public, semi-private* or *private* patient. Unfortunately, you can't mix the type of care you receive. In other words, if you want a private room in one of the public hospitals, you have to be under the private care of a consultant obstetrician — but even then there are no guarantees. . . .

Public Care

Every mum-to-be who lives in Ireland normally is entitled to free maternity care, covering antenatal visits, labour and delivery and postnatal care including home births. When you ring the hospital to make your first appointment, you will be asked if you intend to visit as a public, semi-private or private patient.

If you are a *public* patient, you will attend the hospital's antenatal clinic (or their local clinic in your community). You may see the same doctor on each visit, or you may not — it's pot luck really. Alternatively, if you have a fairly straightforward pregnancy, you can choose the midwives' clinic. You are far less likely to end up with a caesarean or routine intervention at the midwife-led clinic than if you're in the regular maternity ward. Midwife-led care is well documented to be the care of choice for mothers with no complications.

When you come into the hospital to give birth, don't expect your consultant to greet you at the door. The truth is, you may not even see your consultant unless there is a problem. You will labour in one place, then quite often play musical gurneys and move to the delivery ward, then to the public postnatal ward, so pack a light lunch; you'll probably cover quite a bit of mileage. Don't bother with the hospital tour — you'll get to see plenty of it when you're in labour (all joking aside, I highly recommend taking a hospital tour ahead of time). Chances are you will not have met the midwives or doctors who attend your labour and delivery. After the birth of your baby, you will be moved to the public ward for your stay, generally of about three days. A small number of hospitals now offer early discharge schemes, allowing you to go home early from hospital with follow-up care. If you feel you would like to be discharged a few hours after the birth, ask at your first visit if the hospital supports this.

Semi-private and Private Care

If you are attending as a *semi-private patient,* you may see a consultant privately, or attend the semi-private clinic. This clinic is run by the consultant and his/her team. In some hospitals a team member or the doctor on duty at the time may deliver your baby. After delivery, you will stay on a semi-private ward, with approximately 3–5 other mothers.

If you are attending *privately,* you will be assigned your very own consultant who you will most likely get to see at each of your appointments; you can request a particular doctor. Your consultant may not necessarily be available to attend your birth. Private care also entitles you to a private room, although, again, this is dependent on availability and as the birth rate continues to grow and hospitals continue to close, I wouldn't get my hopes up. It is also possible to find your own consultant; but do yourself and your baby a favour and don't choose one based on your best friend's experiences or from pregnancy message boards. This is one of the biggest decisions you'll ever make, so take your time and ask questions.

Maternity and Infant Care Scheme

You may opt for services under the Maternity and Infant Care Scheme, which is a system of combined care, split between your GP and a maternity unit/hospital. The MICS service is provided by your GP and a consultant. You don't have to have a medical card to avail of this. Virtually all GPs have agreements with the health boards to provide these services; they do not have to be part of the GPs and medical card system. The scheme also provides for two post-natal visits to your GP. You'll have to get the forms from your GP and send them to your local HSE Area. You may need to follow up on your application.

Your GP provides an initial examination and probably a pregnancy test if you want one, if possible before 12 weeks, and a further six examinations during the pregnancy, which are alternated with visits to the hospital where you're planning on giving birth. The schedule of visits may be changed by your general practitioner and/or hospital obstetrician depending on your individual situation.

Around five extra visits will also be scheduled with your GP if you suffer from high blood pressure or diabetes. Only pregnancy-related complaints are covered at no charge. If you're dying with the 'flu and go to see your GP, it's not covered!

After you have your baby, your GP will examine the baby at two weeks and both you and baby at six weeks.

In certain circumstances, where a mother opts for a home birth, the health board will provide a grant of around €1,270 towards midwifery costs. Some health boards have suspended payment of the home birth grant indefinitely; the Home Birth Association can give you more information on these issues.

You are entitled to free in-patient and out-patient public hospital services in respect of the pregnancy and the birth and is not liable for any of the hospital charges.

Infant Care Services

The GP who takes care of you also provides care for your newborn. This includes two free developmental exams during the first six weeks following the birth. Your baby's entitlement to free GP services after that depends on whether you have a medical card. In other words, visits to the GP for any conditions related to the baby's health during this six-week period or afterwards are not covered by the scheme unless the parents have a medical card.

The public health nurse visits you at home during the first six weeks, which is a great incentive for new mums to try and get dressed before 4.00 pm!

Pregnancy and Employment Guidelines

Time off work and Antenatal Classes

Section 8 of the Maternity Protection (Amendment) Act 2004 allows you to take paid time off work to attend one set of antenatal classes (but not the last three of the series of classes, as these would normally occur after maternity leave has started). This entitlement is for *one* set of classes across *all* pregnancies while in employment. So, if you use your full entitlement, say, for your first baby, you don't get time off next around. If for any reason you are unable to attend some classes due to reasons beyond your control (e.g. pregnancy complications) you can carry over your entitlement to paid time off work to attend any untaken classes to your subsequent pregnancies (except the last three in a set).

Here's an example: you are attending a set of eight classes and this is your first pregnancy in employment. You are only entitled to be paid while attending five of those classes (as the other three would occur while you are on maternity leave). If for example, you become ill and cannot attend all five classes this time, you may carry over your entitlement to your subsequent pregnancies.

Dads get to come too! Fathers get to take time off to attend the last two antenatal classes immediately prior to the birth.

We all know that not all employers will share your joy about your upcoming birth and impending motherhood! So to keep the peace you're required to notify your employer in writing at least two weeks before classes commence, outlining the dates and times of the classes.

If you do work for a David Brent, he could ask you for evidence of the classes (dates, times, etc.). If that's the case, I'd make sure to give him a play-by-play explanation of what a bloody show is and how terrible episiotomy is — he'll probably avoid you like the plague after that!

Employment and Antenatal Visits

If you become pregnant while in employment you are entitled, under employment law, to take time off to attend antenatal appointments. Similarly, you are entitled to time off for medical visits after the birth.

Let your employer know in writing about your pregnancy and if possible give him plenty of notice that you'll need time off to attend antenatal appointments.

If this notice is not given for reasons outside your control, then you can retain your entitlement, provided you write to your employer with an explanation and with the notice. You will need to do this within one week of the appointment. For any visit after the first appointment your employer may ask to see your appointment card. (Feels like being back in school!)

You are entitled to medical visits after the birth of your baby for 14 weeks following the birth, including any period taken on maternity leave following the birth.

Breastfeeding and Employment

Under Section 9 of the Maternity Protection (Amendment) Act 2004, certain women in employment who are breastfeeding are entitled to take time off work each day in order to breastfeed. The provision applies to all women in employment who have given birth within the previous six months. Employers are not obliged to provide facilities in the workplace to facilitate breastfeeding if the provision of such facilities would give rise to considerable costs. At the choice of her employer, the woman may therefore opt to:

- Breastfeed in the workplace or express breast milk, where facilities are provided in the workplace by the employer;

- Have their working hours reduced (without loss of pay) to facilitate breastfeeding where facilities are not made available.

Women who are in employment and are breastfeeding are entitled to take one hour (with pay) off work each day as a breastfeeding break. This time may be taken as:

- One 60 minute break

- Two 30 minute breaks

- Three 20 minute breaks

You should note that breaks may be *longer* and *more frequent* if agreed between the woman and her employer. Part-time workers are also entitled to breastfeeding breaks, calculated on a pro-rata basis.

Women who wish to exercise their rights to breastfeed in employment must notify their employer (in writing) of their intention to breastfeed at work. You must confirm this information at least four weeks before the date you intend to return to employment from maternity leave.

Employers can require the employee to supply the child's birth certificate (or some other document confirming the child's date of birth).

MATERNITY LEAVE

Maternity leave is *not* a "baby holiday", as my husband once remarked; it is time to help you recuperate, adjust to motherhood and bond with your new baby. It's a time you will look back on with fondness (those mornings spent cooing over your little one) or with horror (those days when getting showered by the time your hubby got home so you could prove how great you were doing was the highlight of your day). Some women complain that maternity leave goes by too quickly and others can't wait to get back to work, if only to have conversations that don't revolve around the colour of bowel movements and nipple confusion.

If you become pregnant while in employment in Ireland, you are entitled to take *maternity leave* for 22 weeks (in 2007 it goes up to 26 weeks, with the option of 16 weeks' additional unpaid leave). At present, at least two weeks have to be taken before the end of the week of your baby's expected birth and at least four weeks after. You can decide how you would like to take the remaining twelve weeks. Generally, employees take four weeks before the birth and 14 weeks after. (Unfortunately, it's not just a rumour that some midwives may tweak dates so the mother can work right up until her due date. So instead of our legislation being forced to become more family-friendly, we are allowing it to become less family-friendly.)

The entitlement to maternity leave from employment extends to all female employees in Ireland (including casual workers), regardless of how long you have been working for the organisation or the number of hours worked per week. However, you do have to fulfil certain conditions before you are eligible to be paid for maternity leave — see below.

You are also entitled to take up to a further eight weeks' unpaid maternity leave. If you can afford it and aren't going demented adjusting to motherhood, take it.

You must give your employer at least four weeks' written notice of your intention to take maternity leave. Get a medical certificate confirming your pregnancy. If you intend to take the additional eight weeks' maternity leave you must provide your employer with at least four weeks' written notice. Put everything in writing so there's no confusion or questions later.

It's not a bad idea to keep in touch with your employer while you're on maternity leave and you need to give him at *least four weeks' written notice* of your return date.

Public Holidays and Annual Leave

You are entitled to leave for any public holidays that occur during your maternity leave (including additional maternity leave). The right of employees to leave for public holidays is set down in Section 21 of the Organisation of Working Time Act, 1997.

Maternity Leave and Annual Leave

Time spent on maternity leave (including additional maternity leave) is treated as though you've never left the office, so you can still accrue holidays.

Stillbirths and Miscarriages

If you have a stillbirth or miscarriage any time after the 24th week of pregnancy, you are still entitled to full maternity leave. This means a basic period of 18 weeks and also eight weeks additional maternity leave. If you have satisfied the PRSI requirements, maternity benefit is payable for the 18 weeks of the basic maternity leave.

Postponing Maternity Leave

You can postpone your maternity leave in strict circumstances — that is, if your baby is hospitalised (not because it's the final week of *Big Brother*!). This right to postpone leave applies whether you are on paid maternity leave or on additional unpaid maternity leave. The maximum amount of time the leave can be postponed for is six months. You must notify your employer as soon as possible if you wish to postpone your maternity leave. Note that your employer has the right to refuse your application to postpone your maternity leave. The catch is that you have to have already taken 14 weeks' maternity leave first, four of which must have been taken after the birth.

If you postpone your maternity leave and return to work, then you may take your leave in one bloc, not later than seven days after your baby has been sent home from hospital. Again your employer can ask you for proof of hospitalisation and discharge after treatment.

If you postpone your maternity leave and return to employment, you need to notify the Department of Social and Family Affairs of this. You must notify them in writing that your child has been hospitalised and you have returned to employment. A letter from your GP/hospital is required to confirm to the Department that the child has been discharged from hospital and your maternity benefit should resume.

Make sure your Personal Public Service Number (PPS) Number is on every document.

Remember, you may only apply to postpone your maternity leave if the baby has been hospitalised.

Illness while on Postponed Maternity Leave

If you have postponed your maternity leave and become ill when you return to work (before resuming your postponed leave), you may be considered to have started your resumed leave on the first day of your absence because of illness. Alternatively, you can choose to have your leave treated as sick leave.

Returning to Work

Yes, that day comes around for most of us! You are entitled to return to work after maternity leave and it can be hard on many parents. Your job is protected and if there have been changes while you've been away your employer must provide you with a suitable alternative. This new position should be reasonably similar to the one you left before materntiy leave.

You are entitled to be treated as if you had been at work during your entire maternity leave. Your employment conditions cannot be worsened by the fact that you have taken maternity leave, and if pay or other conditions have improved while you have been on maternity leave, then you are entitled to these benefits when you return to work.

MATERNITY BENEFIT

Maternity benefit is a payment made to women in Ireland on maternity leave from work and who have paid a certain amount of PRSI. You need to apply for the payment six weeks before you intend to go on maternity leave (16 weeks if you are self-employed). The amount of money paid to you each week will depend on your earnings. If you are already on certain social welfare payments then you will receive half-rate maternity benefit.

Maternity benefit is paid directly to you on a weekly basis into your bank or building society account. Some employers will continue to pay an employee, in full, while you are on maternity leave and require you to remit any social welfare payment to them. You should check your contract of employment to see what applies to you. Maternity benefit is a tax-free payment. If for any reason your claims are refused you can always appeal the decision.

Leave Certification

All employees must have their leave certified by their employer. However, if you get a P45 within 14 weeks of your estimated due date and you've satisfied the PRSI contribution conditions, benefit will be payable from the day after the date on the P45.

Length of Time Maternity Benefit is Paid

Maternity benefit is paid for 22 weeks. At least two weeks and not more than 14 weeks' leave must be taken before the end of the week in which your baby is due. If your baby is born later than expected and you have less than four weeks' maternity leave left, you may be entitled to extend your maternity leave to ensure that you have a full four weeks off following the week of the birth. In these circumstances, maternity benefit will continue to be paid to you until the baby is four weeks old. You need to notify social welfare by sending them a letter from your GP stating the date on which your baby was born.

If your baby is born prematurely before your scheduled period of maternity leave has begun, get your doctor to send a letter to social welfare (Maternity Benefit Section).

If you are employed you must have:

- At least 39 weeks' PRSI paid in the 12-month period before the first day of your maternity leave; *or*

- At least 39 weeks' PRSI paid since first starting work and, in general, at least 39 weeks PRSI paid or credited in the second last complete tax year before the year in which your maternity leave commences. (So if you are going on maternity leave in May 2006, the relevant tax year is 2004. If a tax year later than the relevant tax year has ended before the start of your maternity leave (in this case 2005), contributions in that tax year may be used to help you qualify for maternity benefit. Confusing, eh?); *or*

- At least 26 weeks' PRSI paid in the relevant tax year and at least 26 weeks PRSI paid in the tax year prior to the relevant tax year.

If you are self-employed you must have:

- 52 weeks' PRSI contributions paid at Class S in the relevant tax year before the year in which your claim is made; *or*

- 52 weeks' PRSI contributions paid at Class S in the tax year prior to the relevant tax year before the year in which your claim is made; *or*

- 52 weeks' PRSI contributions paid at Class S in the tax year later than the relevant tax year.

If you are now self-employed but you were in insurable employment before you became self-employed, the PRSI contributions (Class A, E and H) paid by you in that employment may help you qualify for maternity benefit if you do not satisfy the self-employment conditions as stated above.

If you are already on a payment, half-rate maternity benefit is payable if you are getting any one of the following payments:

- One-Parent Family Payment

- Widow's (Contributory) Pension

- Widow's (Non-Contributory) Pension

- Deserted Wife's Benefit

- Prisoner's Wife's Allowance

- Orphan's (Contributory) Allowance

- Orphan's (Non-Contributory) Pension

- Death Benefit by way of Widow's/Widower's or Dependent Parents' Pension (under the Occupational Injuries Scheme)

For new claimants, payment of the half-rate Child Dependant Allowance will be discontinued where a recipient's spouse's weekly income is more than €300.

Insurance from Employment in Another Country

If you were previously employed in a country covered by EU Regulations, and you were paying social insurance, you may have your insurance record in that country added to your Irish PRSI contributions provided that you have paid at least one full-rate PRSI contribution since your return to Ireland.

Disqualification from Maternity Benefit

Maternity Benefit will be stopped if you engage in any other work other than domestic activities in your own home.

Rates: How Much Am I Entitled To?

If you are employed, your weekly rate of Maternity Benefit is calculated by dividing your gross income in the relevant tax year by the number of weeks you actually worked in that year — 80 per cent of this amount is payable weekly. The relevant tax year is the second last complete income tax year before the year in which your maternity leave starts.

If you are self-employed, your weekly rate of maternity benefit is calculated by dividing your gross income in the relevant tax year by 52 weeks — 80 per cent of this amount is payable weekly, subject to a minimum payment and a maximum payment.

CONTACTS

For all information relating to government entitlements, visit http://www.oasis.gov.ie/birth/ Also, see the booklet *Employment Rights Explained*, Comhairle, 2003, a useful free booklet providing lots of information on employment rights, including a section on Maternity and Adoptive Leave.

The Equality Authority has responsibility for overseeing the implementation of the maternity leave legislation in Ireland. Queries about your entitlement to maternity leave, postponing leave, etc. should be addressed to: The Equality Authority, Clonmel Street, Dublin 2; Tel: 01-4173333; Fax: 01-4173366; E-mail: info@equality.ie

If you wish to apply for maternity benefit, you should contact: The Department of Social and Family Affairs, Maternity Benefit Section, Government Buildings, Ballinalee Road, Longford; Tel: 043-45211 or 01-8748444.

GLOSSARY

Active Management of Labour: Protocol for managing the birth process through intervention, designed by the National Maternity Hospital in Dublin

Amniotic Fluid: The clear fluid that your baby floats in during pregnancy

Amniotomy: See ARM

Apgar Score: A scoring system that evaluates the newborn's well-being

ARM (Artificial Rupture of Membranes): Membranes are released artificially with an amniohook (looks like a crochet hook) instead of spontaneously

Auscultation: To listen to your baby's heartbeat

Bedrest: Confinement to bed on medical advice

Birth Plan: A written document to help you to define your birth preferences with your caregiver

Birthing Ball: A large plastic ball that you can use during labour as a comfort measure (also known as an exercise ball or yoga ball)

Bishops Score: A system of points that may indicate the success of an induction

Braxton Hicks: Sporadic tightening/hardening of the uterus (also known as warm-up or practice labour)

Breaking the Waters: See ARM

Breech: A baby that is presenting feet or backside first

Caesarean Section: method of delivering a baby surgically through the abdomen

Cardiotogography (CTG): A machine that monitors baby's heart rate

Catheter: a thin tube that is inserted into the urethra to drain the bladder when you have an epidural

Cervix: The opening to the uterus

Colic: A term associated with fussy babies that tend to have crying bouts in the evening for several hours

Colostrum: An important nutrient- and antibody-rich liquid that is present in your breasts before your milk "comes in"

Contraction: Tightening of the uterine muscles

Cord Clamping: Restriction of the blood from the placenta to your baby by a device (clamp) after the third stage of labour

CPD (Cephalopelvic Disproportion): A rare condition where the baby cannot be born vaginally due to the position/size of your baby and or due to malformation of the mothers pelvis

Dilation: The process of the cervix opening from 0 cm to 10 cm

Directed/Coached Pushing: Being instructed how to push (not mother-led)

Domino Scheme: Community midwife-run scheme that encourages home birth and early release from hospital (short for "Domicillary In and Out")

Doppler: A device for listening to your baby's heartbeat

Doula: A trained labour companion clinically proven to reduce caesarean rates

Eclampsia: The occurrence of seizures not attributed to another cause during pregnancy, usually after the twentieth week

EDD: Estimated Due Date

Entonox: A combination of gas and air used for pain relief in labour

Epidural: A method of pain relief produced by an injection into the spine

Episiotomy: A surgical cut to the perineal area to enlarge the vaginal opening

Evidence Based Care: Practices that are based on the best available clinical research

Expectant Management of Labour: A philosophy of care that adopts a wait-and-see attitude instead of routinely intervening in the normal process of birth

External Cephalic Version (ECV): A technique to manually turn a breech baby to a vertex position

Fetoscope: A device used to monitor your baby's heart rate

Foetal Distress: Reduction of oxygen to the baby, often indicated by consistent irregular heart rate

Foetal Ejection Reflex: The biologically normal spontaneous birth reflex which expels the baby, most commonly seen in an undisturbed birth

Foetal Monitoring: A method of determining the well-being of the baby

Forceps: An obstetric instrument used in assisted deliveries

Forewater Leak: Leak of the amniotic fluid in front of the presenting part of the baby

Guthrie (Heel) Test: Screening test on newborns to detect PKU

Hindwater Leak: Amniotic fluid that releases from an area other than the presenting part (membranes can spontaneously repair themselves)

Hypertension: High blood pressure

HypnoBirthing: An antenatal programme focused on relaxation and visualisation for birth

Induction: The process of artificially starting labour

Kangaroo Care: A way of holding a premature baby so that there is skin-to-skin contact

Kegels: Exercises to tone and strengthen the pelvic floor muscles

Labour — First Stage: Loosely defined as the initial stages of labour when the cervix dilates to 10 cm

Labour — Second Stage: The birth of your baby

Labour — Third Stage: Delivery of the placenta

Lactation Consultant: A professional trained in breastfeeding support

Lithotomy: The "on your back" birth position

Lotus Birth: The process of leaving the cord attached to the placenta and baby for several days

Meconium: A bowel movement that happens in utero or in the early days following birth

Membrane Sweep: A method of induction

Midwife: Caregiver specialising in normal birth

MLU: Midwife Led Unit

Moxibustion: A holistic therapy using heat and herbs, used to turn a breech baby

Multip: A woman who has given birth before

Obstetrician: A caregiver specialising in abnormal and surgical birth

Oxytocin: A hormone generated by the brain that instructs the uterus to contract

Pelvic Floor: The set of muscles and ligaments that support the uterus

Pethidine: A narcotic drug used in labour for pain relief

Pinard: A tool for manually checking heartbeat intermittently (looks like a little trumpet)

Pitocin: A synthetic hormone used to induce or speed up labour

PKU: An inherited genetic disorder that, if untreated, can cause mental retardation

Placenta Abruption: A serious complication where the placenta comes away from the wall of the uterus prematurely

Placenta Previa: A complication where the placenta covers the cervix

Placenta: An organ that develops in the uterus which draws nourishment in for the baby and takes waste from the baby

PND: Post Natal Depression

Pre-eclampsia: A disorder that occurs only during pregnancy and the postpartum period and affects both the mother and the unborn baby. Swelling, sudden weight gain, headaches and changes in vision are important symptoms.

Primip: A woman who is giving birth for the first time

Prodromal Labour: Normal pre-labour contractions before your labour really gets established

Prolapse (cord): Complication, often caused by ARM, where the cord comes before the baby and is compressed, possibly resulting in foetal distress and caesarean.

Prostaglandin: Hormone that stimulates labour (can be used for induction)

Psycho Prophylactics: Breathing techniques

"Rooming In": Keeping your baby with you at the hospital

Rubella: German measles

"Show": One of the many indicators that your body is preparing for birth; usually accompanied by some blood-tinged mucous

"Skin-to-Skin" Caesarean: A new approach to caesareans to make the experience more gentle for the mother and baby

Sonicaid: A handheld electronic tool to check baby's heart rate

Speculum: A plastic or metal instrument used to separate the walls of the vagina during a gynaecological exam

Swaddle: A method of calming a baby by wrapping him in a light cloth

Syntometrine (aka Ergometrine, Syntocinon, Synthetic Hormone Oxytocin): Used to deliver the placenta in a managed third stage.

TENS (Transcutaneous Electrical Nerve Stimulation): Device used for pain management in labour

Toxemia: see Pre-eclampsia

Transition: The point in labour when the cervix is between 8 and 10 cm dilated, where mothers often experience a lack of confidence

Transverse lie: Your baby is lying horizontally

Ultrasound: The use of ultrasonic waves for diagnostic and monitoring purposes for your developing baby

Umbilical Cord: A cordlike structure that attaches the baby to the placenta carrying oxygen and nutrients to the baby and waste way from the baby to the placenta

Uterus: A hollow muscular organ located in the pelvic cavity of female mammals in which the fertilised egg implants and develops (also known as the womb)

Valsalva: A method of directed pushing by caregivers

VBAC: Vaginal Birth After Caesarean (i.e. for subsequent births)

Ventouse/Vacuum: An obstetric tool used for assisted deliveries

Vertex: Position of baby is head down

Water Birth: The birth of a baby in water

Resources

Ante-Natal Classes: throughout Ireland.

Autism Support

Irish Society for Autism: 16 O'Connell Street Lower, Dublin 1; Tel: 01-8744684; Fax: 01 8744224; E-mail: autism@isa.iol.ie.

Baby Massage

http://www.babymassageireland.com/ Cork mobile: 086-1502136; Dublin mobile: 087-7557536.

Bereavement Support

Bereaved Parents Association, St Francis Day Hospital, Grange Road, Dublin 5; Tel: 01-8318788.

Irish Sudden Infant Death Association, 4 North Brunswick Street, Dublin 7; Tel: 1850 391391; General Enquiries: 01-8732711.

The Miscarriage Association of Ireland, Carmichael Centre, North Brunswick Street, Dublin 7; Tel: 01-8735702. Fax: 8735737.

Birth Pool Hire

Padraicín Ní Mhurchú, 36 Springlawn Court, Blanchardstown, Dublin 15; Tel: 01-8206940.

Naomi Clarkin, Brackloon, Westport, Co Mayo; Tel: 098-50830; Mobile: 086-3495728; E-mail: nomeandkillian@eircom.net.

Ray Thompson, 3 Carraig Mhor, Lott Lane, Kilcoole, Co Wicklow; Tel: 01-2872729.

Máire Reagan, 18 Fairgrove Dr., Bishopstown, Cork; Tel: 021-4342649.

Leslie Boal, Pinnhill House, Gortlee, Letterkenny, Co. Donegal; Tel: 074-26103.

Sarah Barry, Greenmount, Rathmore, Naas, Co. Kildare; Tel: 045-862048.

Birth Trauma Support

Anne Gill: Tel: 01-8450698.

Benig Mauger: www.soul-connections.com

Breastfeeding

La Leche League: http://homepage.eircom.net/~lalecheleague/help.html

Breastfeeding Clinic: www.breastfeeding-clinic.com. Enquiries to eileenosullivan@breastfeeding-clinic.com

www.ilca.org/ — for referrals to lactation consultants in Ireland

www.kellymom.com

Cuidiu (see below)

Cuidiu, The Irish Childbirth Trust

Cuidiu, Carmichael House, Brunswick Street, Dublin 7; Tel: 01-8724501, www.cuidiu-ict.ie

Caesarean Support

ICAN: www.ican-online.org

ICAN Dublin chapter: Tracy Donegan, Tel: 087-0572500

Caesarean Support Group: 111 Wedgewood Maples, Sandyford, Dublin 16. Tel: 01-2954953

Sligo Caesarean Support Group: Gwen Scarbrough (Midwife); Tel: 087-6710985; www.informedbirthireland.com

Vaginal Birth after Caesarean: www.vbac.com

Domino/Home Birth Schemes

Contact the Community Midwives at the National Maternity Hospital, Tel: 01-6373100 or 01-6373177; or your local hospital.

Doulas

Association of Irish Doulas: www.DoulaAssociationofIreland.com

Doula Ireland: www.doulaireland.com; Tracy Donegan, Tel: 087-0572500.

Doula Information (UK): www.doula.org.uk
Doula Information (US): www.DONA.org

Down's Syndrome Support

Down's Syndrome Association of Ireland: Island View Quay Road,
 Rush, Co. Dublin. Tel: 01-8439036

General Pregnancy/Parenting Websites

www.rollercoaster.ie
www.eumom.ie
www.thebabyorchard.com
www.mothering.com
www.babycenter.com
www.magicmum.com

Home Birth

The Homebirth Association of Ireland, 36 Springlawn Court,
 Blanchardstown, Dublin 15; www.homebirth.ie; Tel: 01-8206940;
 E-mail: homebirth@eircom.net.

Holistic Practitioners

www.holisto.com
www.homeopathyireland.net

HypnoBirthing

HypnoBirthing: www.HypnoBirthIreland.com (Tracy Donegan)
www.hypnobirthing.co.uk — for a list of local practitioners

Informed Choices

www.infochoice.org
www.maternitymatters.org
www.motherfriendly.org/
www.aims.org.uk/
www.cochrane.org

Lotus Birth

www.birthlove.com

Midwife-Led Units

Cavan: Tel: 087-9799385

Drogheda: Tel: 087-2584951

Multiple Births

Irish Multiple Births Association: Carmichael House, North Brunswick Street, Dublin 7. Tel: 01 8749056. Email: info@imba.ie

Postnatal Depression

PND Association of Ireland: www.PND.ie; E-mail: support@pnd.ie

Aware, 72 Lower Leeson Street, Dublin 2; Tel: 01-6617211; Telephone helpline: 01-6766166, daily, 10.00 am – 10.00 pm; Fax: (01) 6617217; E-mail: aware@iol.ie

Parentline, Carmichael House, North Brunswick Street, Dublin 7; Tel: 01-8787230; Helpline: 01-8733500; Email: parentline@eircom.net

Mental Health Ireland, Mensana House, 6 Adelaide Street, Dun Laoghaire, Co Dublin; Tel: 01-2841166; E-mail: info@mentalhealthireland.ie

Prenatal Parenting

www.birthpsychology.com

www.prenatalparenting.com

Registering a Birth

General Register Office, Joyce House, 8-11 Lombard Street, Dublin 2; Tel: 01-6354000

Single Parent Support

www.gingerbread.ie

www.solo.ie/

www.treoir.ie

Yoga

www.birthlight.com

www.yogapregnancy.net/

www.yogaireland.com

RECOMMENDED READING

Henci Goer, *The Thinking Woman's Guide to Better Birth*, 1999, Penguin (USA)

Sheila Kitzinger, *The New Pregnancy and Childbirth: Choices and Challenges*, 1980, Michael Joseph, revised editions by Penguin Books

Sears and Sears, *The Pregnancy Book*, 1997, Little, Brown (USA)

Sheila Stubbs, *Birth the Easy Way* (e-book)

Ina May Gaskin, *Ina May's Guide to Childbirth*, 2003, Bantam (USA)

Dr Michel Odent, *The Cesarean*, 2004, Free Association Books, UK

Kim Wildner, *Mothers Intention: How Belief Shapes Birth*, 2003, Harbor and Hill (USA)

Benig Mauger, *Reclaiming the Spirituality of Birth*, 2000, Haling Arts (USA)

Thomas Verny M.D., *Tomorrow's Baby*, 2002, Simon & Schuster (USA)

Granju and Kennedy, Attachment *Parenting: Instinctive Care for Your Baby and Young Child*, 1999 (USA)

Sarah J Buckley, *Gentle Birth, Gentle Mothering*, 2005, One Moon Press (Australia)

Nancy Wainer Cohen, *Open Season*, 1991, Bergin and Garvey (USA)

Suzanne Arms, *Immaculate Deception II*, 2001, Celestial Arts (USA)

INDEX

postnatal depression (PND), 180–3
  how others can help, 183
  preventing, 181–2
  symptoms of, 180
pre-eclampsia, 12, 75, 116
pregnancy, 1, 11–19
  discovering, 11
  employment guidelines, 226–8
  using complementary
    therapies, 57–66
Pregnancy and Childbirth, 5
*Pregnancy, Childbirth and the
  Newborn*, 5, 15
Pregnancy Book, The, 5
premature labour, 71–2
prematurity, 130, 176
prostaglandins, 77
pushing, coached/directed, 56,
  112–13
  risks, 113
pushing stage, 28, 47, 56, 104, 112–
  13, 154

refusal, informed, 35–6
relaxation, 10, 16, 21, 25, 44, 58, 59,
  64, 85, 89, 90–3
rescue remedy, 61
resting during labour, positions
  for, 87–8
"rooming in", 45, 161
Rotunda Hospital, 89
rubella, 13

Schauble, Paul, 92
Sears and Sears, 5
Shanley, Laura, 5–10
"show", 25, 69
showering and bathing (during
  labour), 27, 44, 89, 140

Simkin, Penny, 5, 15
soothers, 45
special care units, 29
speeding up of labour, artificial;
  see augmentation of labour
stem cell collection, 162–3
Stubbs, Sheila, 146–7
swaddling, 186
swelling, 12
syntocinon, 27, 28, 63, 81

taking care of yourself after the
  birth, 178–83
  emotionally, 179–80
  physically, 178–9
Tamaro, Janet, 168
TENS machine, 82
tests, newborn, 165–7
third stage of labour, 111, 161–4
  "managed" versus "natural",
  161–2
toddler adjust to new baby,
  helping, 188–9
twin–twin transfusion syndrome,
  116
twins; *see* multiple births

ultrasound scans, 12, 17–19, 46, 76
  how they work, 18
  safety, 19
  why they are done, 18–19
umbilical cord, 18, 110–11, 126
  clamping, 110–11, 128, 162
  cutting, 9, 56, 128, 155, 162
  prolapsed, 126
  pulsation of, 56, 95, 110
  stem cell collection, 162–4
  wrapped around neck, 49
vaccination, 165–6